Praise for

Blueprints

Clinical Procedures

"I graduated from one of the top medical schools in the country and never received any formal "hand-outs" or training manuals on how to perform such procedures. We did get some hands-on training, but it was limited to suturing and blood-draws—this would have been a heaven send for me in my early clinical years! During my residency training I did receive a handout on some of the procedures covered in this book, but it was downloaded from a website. The problem was it was too text dense, pure paragraph form, difficult to read, and poorly organized. I have not seen any other books that provide the same topics as *Blueprints Clinical Procedures* has, in simple-to-read and easy-to-follow steps."

— *PGY-1 Emergency Medicine Resident, University of California Los Angeles School of Medicine*

"My education on Clinical Procedures included a variety of textbooks, workbooks, and handouts from many different providers in the medical profession. Blackwell's new *Blueprints Clinical Procedures* is beyond one of the best resources I have ever encountered since my initial medical training. The book thoroughly explains every procedure important to the healthcare professional in a uniform manner. Each procedural description is detailed, exact, and well comprehended by any medical provider on any level and it is all in one textbook. *Blueprints Clinical Procedures* is an exciting all-inclusive procedural book that can be used by students and medical providers of all varieties. It is thorough, comprehensive, easily read, and painless to follow."

— *MHS, PA-C, Clinical Coordinator*

"*Blueprints Clinical Procedures* is very handy because it is the one great resource for procedures. The table of contents and how the book is organized into systems is very useful and handy. The information in this book is similar to the directions you would get from residents and attendings, but adds helpful hints and is great for reading before a procedure instead of while or after seeing/doing one."

— *PGY-1, University of North Dakota Family Practice Residency*

"There was little official classroom education on most of these procedures by my medical school so this book was definitely helpful. Often times, medical schools leave procedures out of the classroom and on the wards, but it's hit or miss as to which procedures you'll get to perform, making *Blueprints Clinical Procedures* valuable since you could review the procedures you weren't exposed to."

— *PGY-1 Internal Medicine Resident, University of Colorado School of Medicine*

"*Blueprints Clinical Procedures* is a very good book. I have been looking for such a book since medical school!"

— *PGY-1 Surgery Resident, University of South Alabama Medical Center*

"The templated procedures are helpful because they follow a standard format and "train of thought" employed by virtually every "procedure-oriented" physician. By going through the indication for the procedure and the set-up and equipment needed, it allows the novice reader and the experienced technician to mentally prepare themselves for what will be happening. After seeing a procedure highlighted so well and in a simple step-by-step fashion, I would see no reason why a novice would not be able to perform the listed procedure. The only thing that would hold a student back would be his or her own fears or doubts. *Blueprints Clinical Procedures* surely offers all of the information one would need to feel very confident and comfortable performing each and every procedure listed here."

— *4th year Medical Student, Medical College of Wisconsin*

Blueprints

Clinical Procedures

Laurie L. Marbas, MD, MBA
Resident, Department of Family Medicine
Texas Tech University Health Sciences Center
Lubbock, Texas

Erin Case, MD
Resident, Department of Family Medicine
Texas Tech University Health Sciences Center
Lubbock, Texas

FACULTY ADVISOR
Fiona Prabhu, MD
Assistant Professor, Family and Community Medicine
Texas Tech University Health Sciences Center
Lubbock, Texas
Attending Physician, Family Medicine
Texas Tech University Medical Center
Lubbock, Texas

PHOTOGRAPHER
Michael S. Clement, MD
Fellow, American Academy of Pediatrics
Mountain Park Health Center
Phoenix, Arizona
Clinical Lecturer in Family and Community Medicine
University of Arizona College of Medicine
Consultant, Arizona Department of Health Services

Blackwell
Publishing

Blackwell Publishing, Inc., 350 Main Street, Malden, Massachusetts 02148-5018, USA
Blackwell Publishing Ltd, 9600 Garsington Road, Oxford OX4 2DQ, UK
Blackwell Publishing Asia Pty Ltd, 550 Swanston Street, Carlton, Victoria 3053, Australia

04 05 06 07 5 4 3 2

ISBN: 1-4051-0388-4

        Library of Congress Cataloging-in-Publication Data
Marbas, Laurie L.
    Blueprints clinical procedures / Laurie L. Marbas, Erin Case ; faculty
advisor, Fiona Prabhu ; photographer, Michael S. Clement.
        p. ; cm.
Includes index.
    ISBN 1-4051-0388-4 (pbk.)
    1. Clinical medicine.
    [DNLM: 1. Diagnostic Techniques and Procedures—Handbooks. 2.
Therapeutics—Handbooks. WB 39 M312b 2004] I. Title: Clinical
procedures. II. Case, Erin. III. Title.

    RC48.M37 2004
    616—dc22
                                    2003022939

A catalogue record for this title is available from the British Library

Acquisitions: Beverly Copland
Development: Kate Heinle
Photography: Michael S. Clement, MD
            Mesa, Arizona
Production: Jennifer Kowalewski
Cover design: Hannus Design Associates
Interior design: Leslie Haimes
Typesetter: Peirce Graphic Services, in Stuart, FL
Printed and bound by Walsworth Publishing, in Marceline, MO

For further information on Blackwell Publishing, visit our website: www.blackwellmedstudent.com

NOTICE: The indications and dosages of all drugs in this book have been recommended in the medical literature and conform to the practices of the general community. The medications described do not necessarily have specific approval by the Food and Drug Administration for use in the diseases and dosages for which they are recommended. The package insert for each drug should be consulted for use and dosage as approved by the FDA. Because standards for usage change, it is advisable to keep abreast of revised recommendations, particularly those concerning new drugs.

The publisher's policy is to use permanent paper from mills that operate a sustainable forestry policy, and which has been manufactured from pulp processed using acid-free and elementary chlorine-free practices. Furthermore, the publisher ensures that the text paper and cover board used have met acceptable environmental accreditation standards.

Brief Table of Contents

Informed Consent

Prior to beginning any medical procedure, it is important to obtain an informed consent from the patient that is in line with your institution's legal forms and practices. In fact, consider the informed consent to be an important first step in any intervention performed.

Informed consent is a contract between the caregiver and patient that recognizes the patient's right to be involved in decisions regarding his/her own health care. Furthermore, it is also the duty of the caregiver to provide adequate education to the patient in order for them to make a properly informed decision.

A complete informed consent generally should include a thorough discussion of all of the following elements:

- The patient's condition/diagnosis that warrants the procedure

- The nature of the procedure itself

- The potential benefits yielded by the procedure

- The potential risks associated with the procedure

- Any alternative treatments to the procedure

The patient should then be evaluated for his/her understanding of the discussion, and, lastly, the patient can voluntarily express his/her desire to proceed with the procedure in question. It is important that such a discussion be carried out in lay terms that can be suitably comprehended by the patient.

NOTICE

None of the procedures described in this book should be performed by a medical student without supervision. There are, of course, institutional preferences on the performance of some procedures. In such cases, variations may be specified by the resident or attending physician.

All procedures should be performed in the presence of an upper-level resident or attending physician. Failure to represent yourself as a student physician, as well as unclear or misleading descriptions of your training status can constitute a breach of the informed consent patient-caregiver contract and should be discouraged and avoided. Neither the Publisher nor the editors assume any liability for any injury and/or damage to persons or property arising from this publication.

THE PUBLISHER

About the Authors

Dr. Laurie Marbas grew up in the town of Portales, New Mexico, and is currently a first-year resident in the Family Medicine residency at Texas Tech University Health Sciences Center in Lubbock, Texas. She finished a dual MD/MBA degree while at Texas Tech University Health Sciences Center School of Medicine. She also attended the University of Portland in Portland, Oregon, graduating with a B.S. in Biology.

While in medical school, Dr. Marbas created and authored six books in the Visual Mnemonic Series (VMS) published by Blackwell. VMS books are humorous cartoons that help students memorize facts in subjects such as pharmacology, microbiology, pathology, anatomy and physiology, biochemistry, and behavioral sciences. These cartoons helped her (and her classmates) survive the intense challenges of completing medical school while raising three small children and taking night courses for her MBA degree.

Dr. Marbas' favorite times are those spent with her husband, Patrick, and their three children, Emily, Jonathan, and Gabriel. Her grandmother, Maxine, is also part of the Marbas household and has, thankfully, recovered from a recent bout of cancer. Dr. Marbas is an active member in her church and believes her faith is a cornerstone in her life.

Dr. Erin Case grew up in Smithville, Texas, a small town outside of Austin. As a child, she spent much time along the Colorado River, with her black lab, Bird, and her sister and brother, Gert and Johnny, who were often her closest friends. She attended Southwest Texas State University in San Marcos and later graduated from Stephen F. Austin State University in Nacogdoches, Texas, where she received her undergraduate degree in chemistry with a minor in biology. While in Nacogdoches, she met her husband, Jay, and together they have a beautiful daughter, Violet. As a family, they enjoy backyard barbecues, going to the park, and outdoor excursions.

Dr. Case and Dr. Marbas met on the first day of medical school. Because they were the only mothers in the class, they became instant friends. While co-authoring several books, they survived many personal difficulties and medical school together. Dr. Case is also currently a first-year resident in the Family Medicine Department at Texas Tech University Medical Center in Lubbock, Texas.

Dedication

I would like to dedicate this book to Emily, Jonathan, and Gabriel, three beautiful blessings in my life. Throughout my medical education I have also been blessed with many opportunities, for which I thank the Lord every day. Special appreciation must go to my loving family including my husband, Patrick, and my grandmother, Maxine. I would also like to thank my mother, Patricia Lockridge, for her support and encouragement, and my dad, James Lockridge, and sister, Heather Robinette, for their cheerful volunteering. Another thanks goes to Erin Case for her supportive friendship during this project.

—Laurie

I dedicate this book to all of my beautiful family and friends: my husband, Jay; my sweet potato, Violet; my Mom and Dad, Christine and Roger; Leslie, DuBard, Jess, Sophia, and Baby Rachel; Johnny, Aidan, Autumn, and Stacy; my Gango; Granny Joy and Papa Dan; Todd, Kelly, Seth, and Sydney; Grampa Jerry; Addie Lee Morris; Gen Gen and Noni; Aunt Mary; Wanda and Judy; Joann and Tamara; Nehal Shah; Grady Goodwin; Amy Thompson; Ashis Barad; Elizabeth Kirch; Jan Seddighzadeh. A very special thanks to my superhero, Laurie—I hope I can repay your kindness someday.

—Erin

Table of Contents

HOW TO INTERPRET

APPENDICES

INDEX

Contributors

Laura Baker, MD

Associate Professor
Department of Family and Community Medicine
Texas Tech University Health Sciences Center
Lubbock, Texas

Kelly Bennett, MD

Assistant Professor, Family Medicine
Medical Director, Student Health Services
Texas Tech University Health Sciences Center
Lubbock, Texas

Jason T. Bradley, MD

Cardiology Fellow
Department of Internal Medicine
Texas Tech University Health Sciences Center
Lubbock, Texas

Kellie Flood-Shaffer, MD, FACOG

Assistant Professor, OB/GYN
Texas Tech University Health Sciences Center
Lubbock, Texas
Attending Faculty
Texas Tech University Medical Center
Lubbock, Texas

Calvin Kuo, MD

Resident, Department of Family Medicine
Texas Tech University Health Sciences Center
Lubbock, Texas

Walter A. Lajara-Nanson, MD

Assistant Professor, Neuropsychiatry and Behavioral
Science
Texas Tech University Health Sciences Center
Lubbock, Texas
Attending Physician, Neurologist/Psychiatrist
Texas Tech University Medical Center
Lubbock, Texas

Brent Paulger, MD

Paulger Dermatology
Lubbock, Texas

Jeff W. Paxton, MD

Assistant Professor
Director of Sports Medicine
Department of Family and Community Medicine
Texas Tech University Health Sciences Center
Lubbock, Texas

Kirsten K. Robinson, MD

Resident, Pediatrics
Texas Tech University Health Sciences Center
Lubbock, Texas

Michael D. Shaffer, DO

Chief Resident
Department of Family and Community Medicine
Texas Tech University Health Sciences Center
Lubbock, Texas

Haden Steffek, MD

Resident
Anesthesia Department
Texas Tech University Health Sciences Center
Texas Tech University Medical Center
Lubbock, Texas

David C. Waagner, MD

Associate Professor, Pediatrics
Texas Tech University Health Sciences Center
Chief, Division of Pediatric Infectious Diseases
Texas Tech University Medical Center
Lubbock, Texas

Acknowledgments

We would like to express our deepest thanks to the many people who collaborated with us on this book. We especially thank our contributors for their dedication, assistance, knowledge, and inspiration. A special thanks goes to our models and volunteers, without whom this book would not have been possible.

A debt of gratitude is also owed to our home away from home, the Texas Tech University Health Sciences Center Family Medicine Department, and to Dr. Fiona Prabhu for her role as faculty advisor. A million thanks to Dr. Fred Hagedorn for constant support and encouragement. We also send a great thank-you to Dr. Mike Clement and his wife, Roberta, for their creative talent behind the camera lens.

Finally, we would like to thank Beverly Copland, Kate Heinle, and all the great staff members of Blackwell Publishing for their patience and support throughout the creation of this book.

We would like to thank the following individuals for their support and guidance.

Dr. Dana Fathy

Heather Fathy

"Baby" Fathy

Dr. Jodie "DD" Dejecacion

Conner Dejecacion

Dr. Shane Hord

Rachel Hord

Madison Hord

Dr. Tammy Camp

Dr. Cynthia Jumper

Sandra Caballero, RN, BSN

Claude Lobstein

Penne Richards

Jesse Leal

Mike Lindley

Eric Givens

Nik Matthews

Mae Naron

Scott Frankfather

Dr. Jane Counts (J.C.)

Dr. Courtney Barton

Dr. Jason Hubbard

Dr. Jim Tarpley

Dr. Michelle Kirk

Dr. Adam Gunder

Victor Goff

Dear Reader,

Blueprints Clinical Procedures was created for all health care professionals who perform procedures. Whether you just need a refresher or you've never performed the procedure before, this book will provide the how-to information you need to be prepared.

Here, **in one handy resource,** you will find ALL the procedures you need to know. Detailed, step-by-step instructions are given for nearly 100 procedures, and close to 300 full-color photographs and illustrations are included to visually demonstrate techniques. In this case, a picture *is* worth a thousand words.

Medical students, residents, PAs, NPs, and other health care practitioners will find this an invaluable resource to use while in school and later in practice.

Features

Designed to be extremely valuable, the book provides:

- **Anatomical organization** so you can find the procedure you need quickly

- **Templated procedures** that offer consistent presentation

- **Detailed photos** and drawings that illustrate how to perform the procedures

- **Pearls/Tips boxes** containing critical information such as contraindications, and special "how-to" advice, similar to the information received from residents and attending physicians while on rounds

- **Special *How to Interpret* section** delineates interpretation of ABGs, chest, and abdominal x-rays . . . a vital addition to clinical work

- **Appendices** with important supplemental content

- **Sterile glove icon** next to the title of procedures performed under sterile conditions—reminding you to prepare properly *before* beginning a procedure to prevent the all-too-common mistake of getting halfway through preparations, only to realize that the procedure is sterile and you must start all over

Organization

Sections are arranged by anatomical region so the information you need can be accessed quickly. For example, the venipuncture procedure is found in the "Heart and Peripheral Vasculature" chapter. Two special sections cover performing procedures on pregnant patients and infants and children.

Within each section, procedures use templated headings to help you find what you need:

- **Purpose**—Describes the indications for the procedure

- **Equipment Needed**—Lists all the equipment required, and indicates whether it must be sterile or not

- **Technique**—Details clear, thorough steps on how to perform the procedure

- **Complications**—Explains commonly encountered problems

- **Post-Procedure Care**—Gives guidance on follow-up care and patient education

Appendices

These valuable supplements present specialized information on clinical care, interacting with patients, and proper documentation, specifically:

- Writing progress and procedure notes
- Using the effective "SOAP notes" format
- Taking a complete history while performing a physical
- Helpful Spanish/English History and Physical Terms and Phrases

Blueprints **Clinical Procedures** is a must-have resource that you can keep throughout your medical career. Whether performing a procedure for the very first time, or polishing your technique, this book contains the comprehensive content you need to be accurate and safe.

Please send any comments or suggestions about this book to blue@bos.blackwellpublishing.com

The Publisher
Blackwell Publishing

Abbreviations

A/a	alveolar-arterial oxygen gradient	βHCG	beta human chorionic gonadotropin
ABCs	airway, breathing, circulation	BID	twice a day (bis in die)
ABG	arterial blood gas	BiPAP	bilevel positive airway pressure
AC	before meals (ante cibum)	BOOP	bronchiolitis obliterans-organizing pneumonia
AC	acromioclavicular	BP	blood pressure
ACE	angiotensin-converting enzyme	BPAD	bipolar affective disorder
aCL	anticardiolipin (antibody)	bpm	beats per minute
ACLS	Advanced Cardiac Life Support	BPP	biophysical profile
ACOG	American College of Obstetrics and Gynecology	BPPV	benign paroxysmal positional vertigo
ACTH	adrenocorticotropic hormone	BSA	body surface area
AD	Alzheimer's dementia or disease	BUN	blood urea nitrogen
AFib	atrial fibrillation	BV	bacterial vaginosis
AFB	acid-fast bacilli	BVM	bag valve mask
AFP	alpha-fetoprotein	C&S	culture and sensitivity
AFV	amniotic fluid volume	C-peptide	insulin chain C-peptide
AGCUS	atypical glandular cells of undetermined significance	C-section	cesarean section
AI	amnioinfusion	C-spine	cervical spine
AIDS	acquired immunodeficiency syndrome	CABG	coronary artery bypass graft
ALT	alanine aminotransferase	CaCl$_2$	calcium chloride
ANA	antinuclear antibody	CAD	coronary artery disease
ANCA	antineutrophil cytoplasmic antibody	cap	capsule
AP	anteroposterior	c-ANCA	cytoplasmic antineutrophil cytoplasmic antibody
APS	antiphospholipid syndrome	CBC	complete blood cell count
APSAC	anistreplase, anisoylated plasminogen-streptokinase activator complex	cc	cubic centimeter (for solids and gases but mL for liquids)
APTT	activated partial thromboplastin	CD41	helper T cell (cluster of differentiation no. 41)
ARC	AIDS-related complex	CDC	Centers for Disease Control and Prevention, Atlanta, Ga.
ARDS	adult respiratory distress syndrome		
ARF	acute renal failure	CEA	carcinoembryonic antigen
ASA	acetylsalicylic acid	CFU	colony-forming unit
ASAP	as soon as possible	CHF	congestive heart failure
ASCUS	atypical squamous cells of undetermined significance	Chol	cholesterol
ASO	antistreptolysin O antibody	CIN	cervical intraepithelial neoplasia (1 to 3: mild to severe)
AST	aspartate aminotransferase		
Atg	anti-human thymocyte globulin	CK	creatine kinase
ATN	acute tubular necrosis	CLL	chronic lymphocytic leukemia
AV	arteriovenous; atrioventricular	cm	centimeter
AZT	zidovudine (Azidothymidine)	CMAP	compound muscle action potential
B12	vitamin B12	CMV	cytomegalovirus
BAER	brainstem auditory evoked responses	CNS	central nervous system
BBT	basal body temperature	CO$_2$	carbon dioxide
BCG	bacille Calmette-Guérin	COPD	chronic obstructive pulmonary disease
BCP	birth control pill	CPAP	continuous positive airway pressure
		CPD	cephalopelvic disproportion

CPK	creatine phosphokinase
CPPD	calcium pyrophosphate dihydrate (crystals) (pseudogout)
CPR	cardiopulmonary resuscitation
Cr	creatinine
CRF	chronic renal failure
CRP	C-reactive protein
CSF	cerebrospinal fluid
CST	contraction stress test
CT	computerized tomography
CVA	cerebrovascular accident
CVAT	costovertebral-angle tenderness
CVD	cerebrovascular disease
CVN	central venous nutrition
CVP	central venous pressure
CVS	cardiovascular system
c/w	consistent with
CXR	chest x-ray film or radiograph
D&C	dilatation and curettage
DBP	diastolic blood pressure
DDAVP	1-deamino-8-D-arginine vasopressin
DDC, ddC	dideoxycytidine, zalcitabine, Hivid
DDI, ddI	dideoxyinosine, didanosine
D5W	5% dextrose in water
D4T	stavudine
DHE	dihydroergotamine
DHT	dihydrotestosterone
DIC	disseminated intravascular coagulation
DIP	distal interphalangeal joint
DKA	diabetic ketoacidosis
dl	deciliter
DM	diabetes mellitus
DPL	diagnostic peritoneal lavage
DPT	diphtheria-pertussis-tetanus (vaccine)
DS	double strength
DSM	Diagnostic and Statistical Manual (of Mental Disorders)
dsDNA	double-stranded deoxyribonucleic acid
DTR	deep tendon reflexes
DTs	delirium tremens
DVT	deep venous thrombosis
D/W	dextrose in water
EBV	Epstein-Barr virus
ECC	endocervical curettage
ECF	extracellular fluid
ECG	electrocardiogram
ECMO	extracorporeal membrane oxygenation

ED	emergency department
EDC	estimated date of confinement
EEG	electroencephalogram
EES	erythromycin ethylsuccinate
EGD	esophagogastroduodenoscopy
EIA	enzyme immunoassay
ELISA	enzyme-linked immunosorbent assay
EM	erythema multiforme
EMG	electromyogram
ENG	electronystagmography
ENT	ear, nose, throat
ER	emergency room
ERCP	endoscopic retrograde cholangiopancreatography
ESR	erythrocyte sedimentation rate
ET	endotracheal tube
FB	foreign body
FDA	U.S. Food and Drug Administration
Fe	iron
FENa	fractional excretion of sodium
FEF	forced expiratory flow
FEV1	forced expiratory volume at 1 second
FFP	fresh frozen plasma
FH	family history
FHR	fetal heart rate
FIO$_2$	forced inspiratory oxygen
FSH	follicle-stimulating hormone
FTA	fluorescent treponemal antibody
FTA-ABS	fluorescent treponemal antibody absorption (test)
5-FU	5-fluorouracil
F/U	follow-up (study, exam, test, care)
FUO	fever of unknown origin
g	gram
G6PD	glucose-6-phosphate dehydrogenase
GBS	group B Streptococcus bacteria, or group B streptococcal infection
GC	gonococcus
GCS	Glasgow Coma Scale
GCT	glucose challenge test
GDM	gestational diabetes mellitus
GE	gastroesophageal
GFR	glomerular filtration rate
GI	gastrointestinal
GM-CSF	granulocyte-macrophage colony-stimulating factor
GN	glomerulonephritis
GnRH	gonadotropin-releasing hormone
GODM	gestational onset diabetes mellitus
gtt	drops (guttae)

GTT	glucose tolerance test	ISA	intrinsic stimulating activity
GU	genitourinary	ITP	idiopathic thrombocytopenia purpura
GXT	graded exercise stress test	IU	International Unit
GYN	gynecologic	IUD	intrauterine device
h, hr	hour	IUFD	intrauterine fetal demise
H&P	history and physical examination	IUGR	intrauterine growth retardation
HA	headache	IUP	intrauterine pregnancy
Hb	hemoglobin	IV	intravenous
HC/AC	head circumference-to-abdominal circumference (ratio)	IVC	inferior vena cava
		IVDA	intravenous drug abuser
HCG	human chorionic gonadotropin	IVP	intravenous pyelogram
HCT	hematocrit	JRA	juvenile rheumatoid arthritis
HCTZ	hydrochlorothiazide	JVD	jugular venous distension
HDL	high-density lipoprotein	JVP	jugular venous pressure
HELLP	hemolysis, elevated liver enzymes, and low platelet count (syndrome)	kg	kilogram
		K, K1	potassium
HepBsAg	hepatitis B surface antigen	KOH	potassium hydroxide
HGE	human granulocytic ehrlichiosis	KS	Kaposi's sarcoma
HIV	human immunodeficiency virus	LA	lupus anticoagulant
HME	human monocytic ehrlichiosis	LAT	preparation of lidocaine, epinephrine (adrenaline), tetracaine
HMG	human menopausal gonadotropin		
h/o	history of	LBBB	left bundle branch block
HPF	high-power field	LDH	lactate dehydrogenase
HRT	hormone replacement therapy	LDL	low-density lipoprotein
HS	at bedtime (hora somni)	LE	lupus erythematosus
HSV	herpes simplex virus	LES	lower esophageal sphincter
ht, Ht	height	LFT	liver function tests
HTN	hypertension	LGI	lower GI (gastrointestinal)
HUS	hemolytic uremic syndrome	LH	luteinizing hormone
HZV	herpes zoster virus	LLQ	left lower quadrant
I&D	incision and drainage	LMP	last menstrual period
I&O	intake and output	LMW	low molecular weight
ICF	intracellular fluid	LOC	loss of consciousness
ICP	intracranial pressure	LP	lumbar puncture
ICU	intensive care unit	LR	lactated Ringer's solution
ID	infectious disease	L/S	lecithin-to-sphingomyelin (ratio)
IDDM	insulin-dependent diabetes mellitus	LSIL	low-grade squamous intraepithelial lesion
IFA	immunofluorescence assay	LUQ	left upper quadrant
IgG	immunoglobulin G	LV	left ventricular
IHSS	idiopathic hypertrophic aortic stenosis	MAI/MAC	Mycobacterium avium-intracellulare/M. avium complex
IM	intramuscular		
IMV	intermittent mandatory ventilation	MAO	monoamine oxidase
IN	intranasally	MAOI	monoamine oxidase inhibitors
INH	isoniazid, isonicotinic acid hydrazide	MAST	military antishock trousers
INR	International Normalized Ratio	MCP	metacarpophalangeal joint
IO	intraosseous	MCV	mean corpuscular volume
IPPV	intermittent positive-pressure ventilation	MDD	major depressive disorder

MDI	metered dose inhaler	PCA	patient-controlled analgesia
MEE	middle ear effusion	PCN	penicillin
mEq	milliequivalent	PCOD	polycystic ovarian disease
mg	milligram	PCP	Pneumocystis pneumonia
μg	microgram	PCR	polymerase chain reaction
MI	myocardial infarction	PCWP	pulmonary capillary wedge pressure
min	minute	PD	Parkinson's disease
mm Hg	millimeters of mercury	PDA	patent ductus arteriosus
mmol	millimole	PE	physical examination
MMPI	Minnesota Multiphasic Personality Inventory	PE	pulmonary embolism
MMR	measles-mumps-rubella (vaccine)	PEEP	positive end-expiratory pressure
MMSE	Mini-Mental State Examination	PEFR	peak expiratory flow rate
mOsm	milliosmole	PET	positron emission tomography
MR	measles and rubella (vaccine)	PFTs	pulmonary function tests
MRI	magnetic resonance imaging	PG	phosphatidylglycerol
MS	multiple sclerosis	pH	hydrogen-ion concentration; pH 7, normal; less is acidic; more is alkaline (or basic)
MTP	metatarsophalangeal joint		
MVP	mitral valve prolapse	PICC	peripherally inserted central catheter
N&V	nausea and vomiting	PID	pelvic inflammatory disease
NCS	nerve conduction study	PIH	pregnancy-induced hypertension
NCV	nerve conduction velocity	PIP	proximal interphalangeal joint
NG	nasogastric	plt	platelet
NHL	non-Hodgkin's lymphoma	PMNs	polymorphonuclear lymphocytes
NIDDM	non-insulin dependent diabetes mellitus	PMS	premenstrual syndrome
NPH	neutral protamine Hagedorn	PO	per mouth (per os)
NPO	nothing by mouth (nulla per os)	pO_2	oxygen partial pressure
NS	normal saline solution	POD	postoperative day
NSAID	nonsteroidal anti-inflammatory drug	PPD	protein purified derivative
NST	nonstress test	PR	per rectum
NSVD	normal spontaneous vaginal delivery	PRN	as needed (pro re nata)
NTD	neural tube defect	PROM	premature rupture of membranes
NTG	nitroglycerin	PSA	prostate specific antigen
O&P	ova and parasites	PSVT	paroxysmal supraventricular tachycardia
OA	osteoarthritis	PT	prothrombin time
OCD	obsessive-compulsive disorder	PTCA	percutaneous transluminal coronary angioplasty
OCP	oral contraceptive pill	PTL	premature labor
OM	otitis media	PTSD	post-traumatic stress disorder
OPV	oral poliovirus	PTT	partial thromboplastin time
ORS	oral rehydration solution	PTU	propylthiouracil
osm, Osm	osmole; osmolality	PUD	peptic ulcer disease
OTC	over the counter	PVC	premature ventricular contraction
PA	posteroanterior	QD	every day (quaque die)
PA	pulmonary artery	QHS	"at every bedtime" (quaque hora somni)
PAC	premature atrial contraction	QID	four times per day (quater in die)
PALS	Pediatric Advanced Life Support	QOD	every other day (tertio quoque die)
Pap	Papanicolaou test or smear	RA	rheumatoid arthritis
PAS	para-aminosalicylic acid	RBC	red blood cell

RCA	right coronary artery		TFT	thyroid function test
REM	rapid eye movement		TG	triglycerides
RF	renal failure		TIA	transient ischemic attack
RLQ	right lower quadrant		TIBC	total iron-binding capacity
R/O, r/o	rule out		TM	tympanic membrane
ROM	rupture of membranes; range-of-motion		TMP/SMX	trimethoprim-sulfamethoxazole (complex)
RSV	respiratory syncytial virus		ToRCHS	toxoplasmosis, rubella, cytomegalovirus, herpes simplex, syphilis
RUQ	right upper quadrant		TPA	tissue plasminogen activator
SBP	systolic blood pressure		TPN	total parenteral nutrition
SGA	small for gestational age		TRH	thyrotropin-releasing hormone
SL	sublingual		TSH	thyroid-stimulating hormone
SLE	systemic lupus erythematosus		TTP	thrombotic thrombocytopenic purpura
SNAP	sensory nerve action potential		TURP	transurethral prostatectomy
SOB	shortness of breath		U	unit
SQ	subcutaneous		UA	urinalysis
SR	slow release		UGI	upper gastrointestinal (tract)
SROM	spontaneous rupture of membrane		URI	upper respiratory infection
SSRI	selective serotonin reuptake inhibitors		U/S	ultrasound, ultrasonogram, ultrasonography
STD	sexually transmitted disease		UTI	urinary tract infection
SVC	superior vena cava		VFib	ventricular fibrillation
T3	triiodothyronine		VTach	ventricular tachycardia
T4	thyroxine		VBAC	vaginal birth after cesarean section
Tb, TB	tuberculosis		VCUG	voiding cystourethrogram
TBG	thyroxine-binding globulin		VDRL	Venereal Disease Research Laboratories (test)
TBSA	total body surface area		V/Q	ventilation-perfusion ratio
TBW	total body water		VSD	ventricular septal defect
TCA	tricyclic antidepressant		WBC	white blood cell (count)
TEE	transesophageal echocardiography			

I. Sterile Technique

It is important to appreciate the proper method of donning sterile gloves and a sterile gown for your patient's protection as well as your own. These methods are used when scrubbing for surgery or performing a sterile bedside procedure.

There are two primary scrub methods: the time method and the brush-stroke method. The time method involves scrubbing for a predetermined amount of time, and the brush-stroke method requires using a predetermined number of brush-strokes when washing. The preferred method varies among institutions. There is one important principle to remember when scrubbing: **unsterile objects should not be touched once scrubbing has begun; the entire scrubbing process must be repeated if this occurs.**

Scrubbing

Brush-stroke method:

1. Turn on water and regulate flow and temperature.

2. Open scrub brush package and lay aside.

3. Wet hands and arms and perform a pre-scrub wash with detergent to about 2 inches above the elbows.

4. Rinse hands and arms thoroughly, being careful not to touch any unsterile object.

5. Retrieve the sterile brush and file. Moisten the brush to create a lather, and use the file to clean under the fingernails. Fingernails should be cleaned under running water.

6. Discard the file.

7. Produce a lather with the sponge side of the brush and then use the sponge's bristles to scrub under the fingernails with about 30 circular strokes.

8. Consider each finger, hand, and arm as having four planar sides. Each surface should then be scrubbed with about 20 circular strokes. Use the bristle side of the brush for the digits and the sponge side for the hand and arm. Completely scrub the hand and arm (to 2 inches past the elbow) on one side before moving to the other side.

9. Add soap or water to the brush as needed during the scrubbing process.

10. Discard the brush.

11. Rinse hands and arms thoroughly, allowing water to run from the hands to the elbows.

12. Lean forward as you dry your hands and arms with a sterile towel. Do not allow any part of the towel or your hands and arms to touch an unsterile object. Use one end of the towel to thoroughly dry one hand and arm, then use the opposite end of the towel to dry the other hand and arm.

 ## Donning a Surgical Gown

IMPORTANT NOTE: If you touch the outside of the gown while putting it on, it is then contaminated and must be discarded. After scrubbing, the hands and arms are considered contaminated if they fall below the waist or touch the body. Only certain areas are considered sterile after donning the gown: the sleeves (excluding the axillary region), and the front of the gown from the waist to a few inches below the neck opening.

A. Closed cuff method:

1. Pick up the gown in its wrapper. Pull the wrapper's tab away from you and grasp with the hand holding the gown (Figures I-1a, I-1b). Continue this until all four corners have been opened revealing the sterile gown. The gown is folded with inside revealed. Grasp the gown and remove it as shown (Figure I-1c).

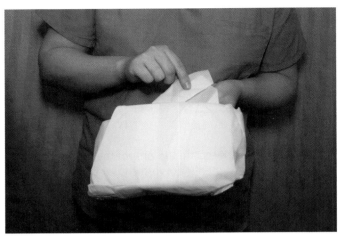

I-1a Opening sterile gown package.

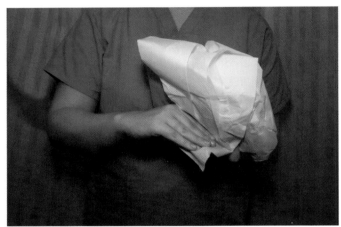

I-1b Tucking paper into hand.

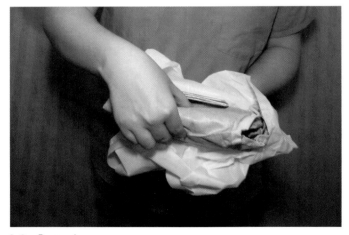

I-1c Removing gown.

2. Grasp the inside shoulder seams and open the gown with armholes facing toward you (Figure I-2). While holding the gown, allow it to fall open without touching any unsterile object (including your body).

3. Slide your arms into the sleeves about 3/4 of the way down.

4. Have an assistant pull the gown up and over your shoulders while you slide your arms to the beginning of the sleeve cuffs and grasp them from the inside to prevent your hands from protruding beyond the sleeve cuff. Have the assistant fasten the back (Figure I-3).

B. Open cuff method:

This procedure is the same as closed cuff, except you do not grasp the inside seam of the sleeve and cuff, but instead allow your hands to partially protrude from the sleeve cuff. You will need an assistant to fasten the back of the gown.

Donning Surgical Gloves

A. Closed cuff method: (This method is preferable because you are less likely to contaminate yourself.)

1. Open sterile gloves and have them ready to pick up before you begin donning the gown.

2. Create a tuck in the cuff of the gown by grasping the material with your hand from within the cuff.

3. Pick up one glove by the folded cuff edge with the sleeve-covered hand (Figure I-4). It may be easier to put on the left glove first if you are right-handed, and vice versa if you are left-handed.

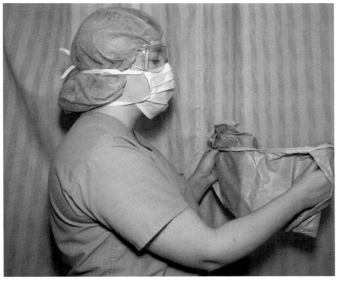

I-2 Grabbing arm folds.

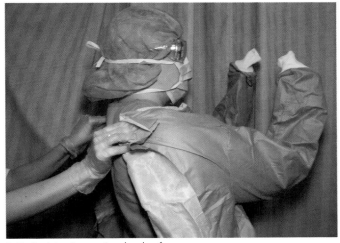

I-3 Assistant securing back of gown.

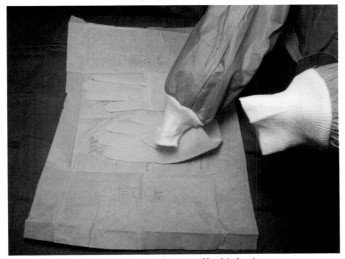

I-4 Closed cuff method: grabbing cuff of left glove.

4. Place the glove on the opposite gown sleeve, palm down, with the glove fingers pointing toward your shoulder. The glove's rolled cuff should be aligned with the seam of the sleeve and cuff (Figure I-5). Your palm should be facing upward and toward the palm of the glove.

5. Hold the glove's bottom rolled cuff-edge with your thumb and index finger.

6. With the opposite hand, grab the glove's uppermost rolled cuff edge and stretch the cuff of the glove over the hand (Figure I-6).

7. Grasp the sleeve cuff and glove cuff and pull the glove onto your hand (Figure I-7).

8. Pull any extra sleeve material from underneath the glove.

9. Put the second glove on using the same method.

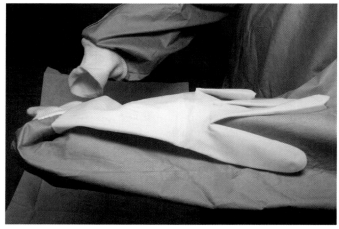

I-5 Closed cuff method: placement of glove on left arm.

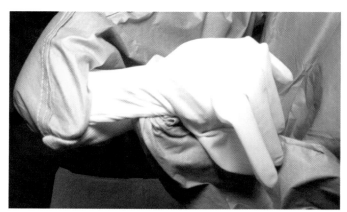

I-6 Closed cuff method: placement of glove onto hand.

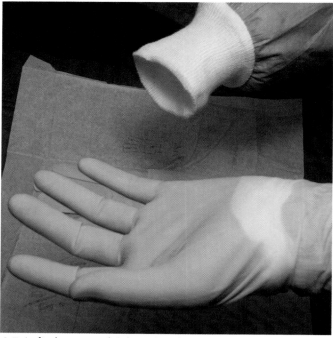

I-7 Left glove completely on hand.

B. Open cuff method:

1. Pick up the sterile glove with your fingertips, making sure you are only manipulating the inside portion of the glove, and slide your opposite hand into the glove (Figure I-8). Be careful not to touch any portion of the sleeve or exterior of the glove with your hand.

2. Release the glove after it has been pulled over the sleeve cuff.

3. Grab the other sterile glove with the already-gloved hand by placing fingers within the fold of the glove (Figure I-9).

4. Stretch the glove over the opposite hand and pull the glove cuff down over the sleeve cuff (Figures I-10a and I-10b).

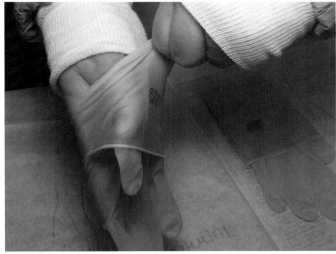

I-8 Open cuff method: placement of glove onto right hand.

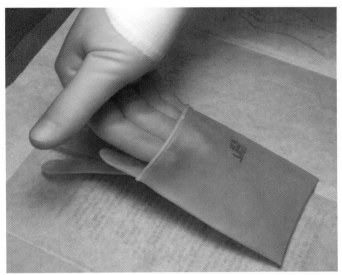

I-9 Open cuff method: placement of second glove.

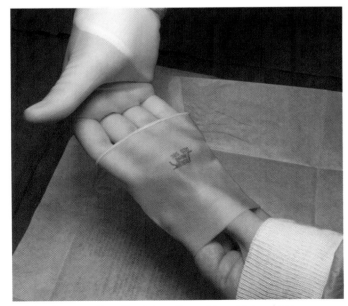

I-10a Open cuff method: insertion of hand into glove.

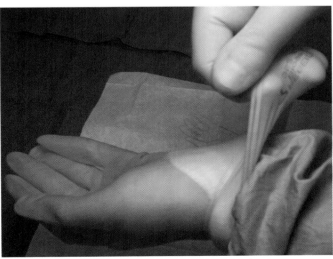

I-10b Open cuff method: securing glove over sleeve.

Final Gown Tie

1. Grasp the paper tab attached to the front of the gown and hand the opposite end to an assistant (Figures I-11a and I-11b).

2. Release the paper tab and turn around in a circle while the assistant remains holding firmly on to the paper tab.

3. Have the assistant securely hold the paper tab as you pull the belt loose from the paper tab and tie it to the belt tie attached to the front of the gown (Figures I-12a and I-12b).

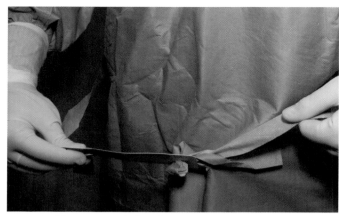

I-11a Pulling paper tab free from gown.

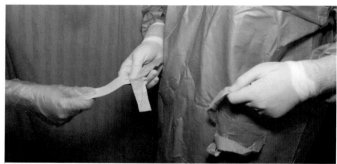

I-11b Handing off paper tab.

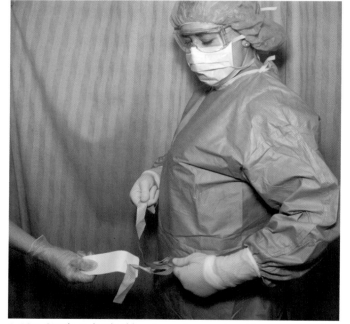

I-12a Sterile individual has turned around and is now removing remaining tie from paper tab.

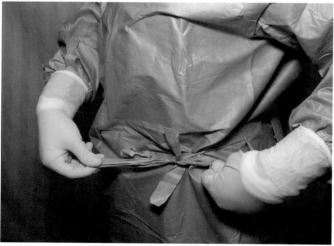

I-12b Securing tie.

Disrobing

A. Reusable cloth gowns:

1. Have an assistant untie the back of the gown and then pull the gown off, leaving the gloves behind.

2. Remove the first glove by grasping the outer surface of one glove, "rubber to rubber" and pull it off (never allowing the outer surface of the glove to touch your skin).

3. Discard the glove.

4. Remove the last glove by placing your fingers inside the cuff of the glove "skin to skin."

5. Discard the glove.

B. Disposable paper gowns:

1. Break the ties by pulling the gown forward, pulling the gloves off as you pull the gown off.

2. Discard the gown and gloves (Figure I-13).

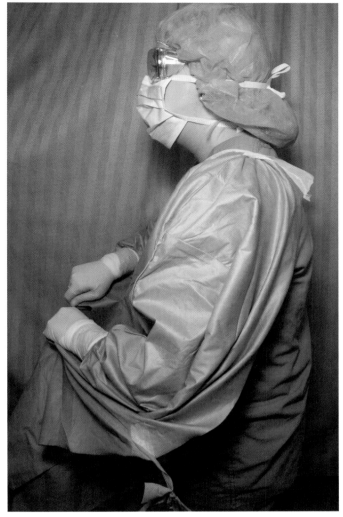

I-13 Gown disrobement.

II. Skin

1. Skin Biopsy

Three common methods of sampling skin are shave biopsy, punch biopsy, and elliptical biopsy. Because many different skin conditions can have similar clinical presentations, a biopsy of the skin for histologic evaluation can aid in the definitive diagnosis of a particular condition. Whenever possible, biopsies should be performed on fresh, well-developed, non-manipulated, and non-excoriated lesions above the knees.

1a. Shave Biopsy

PURPOSE: Useful for elevated lesions when the full thickness of tissue is unimportant. This includes superficial benign lesions such as warts, nevi, seborrheic keratoses, and malignant lesions such as non-melanoma malignancies.

EQUIPMENT NEEDED (FIGURE 1-1):

- Sterile razor blade or No. 15 scalpel blade
- Electrocautery or chemical cautery (Monsel, silver nitrate, or aluminum chloride solution) for hemostasis
- 1% Lidocaine (with epinephrine) for anesthesia
- 3-cc syringe with 22-gauge (or 18-gauge, if preferred) needle to draw up lidocaine
- 30-gauge needle for injection
- Antibiotic ointment
- Self-adhesive bandage
- Alcohol prep pad or povidone iodine (Betadine) cleanser
- Bottle with tissue preservative

TECHNIQUE:

1. Swab the area with alcohol prep pad or Betadine.

2. Inject the base of the lesion intradermally with 0.5–1.5 cc of lidocaine with epinephrine (Figure 1-2). A good intradermal anesthetic result is a white wheal

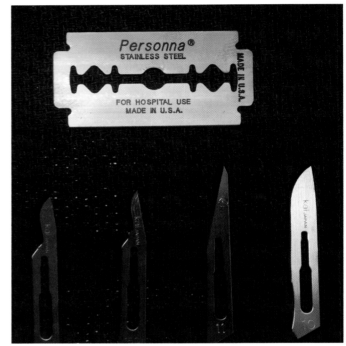

1-1 Blades. Top row (from left to right): flexible Personna blade. Bottom row (from left to right): No. 15, No. 15c, No. 11, and No. 10.

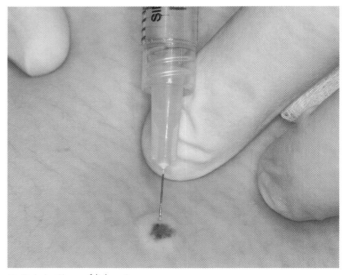

1-2 Injection of lidocaine.

surrounding the lesion. The surrounding tissue is slightly elevated by compression of the tissue between the thumb and index finger (or use sterile forceps for traction).

3. Remove the lesion with a No. 15 blade or, preferably, with a Personna razor blade that can be bent into a curved position (Figure 1-3). Place the blade against the base of the lesion and drawing the blade through the tissue with a cutting/sawing motion.

4. Place the specimen in tissue preservative immediately.

5. Obtain hemostasis with light electrocautery or application of either Monsel or aluminum chloride solution (Figure 1-4).

6. Apply a small amount of antibiotic ointment and cover the wound with a self-adhesive bandage.

COMPLICATIONS:

- Bleeding can occur in patients on aspirin or warfarin, or after the vasoconstrictive effects of the epinephrine wear off.

- Depressed scars or divots can occur. The extent of scarring depends of the depth of the biopsy and the site of the biopsy. Hypertrophic scars can occur on the trunk and proximal extremities.

- Although rare, infection can occur in intertriginous areas or areas heavily colonized with bacteria.

POST-PROCEDURE CARE:

Ask patients to follow the instructions listed below for wound care.

1. Leave the original bandage in place for 24 hours, then clean wound once or twice daily with soap and water or hydrogen peroxide.

2. Apply a layer of bacitracin or bacitracin-polymyxin B ointment, or petroleum jelly to the area.

3. Cover with self-adhesive bandage (optional).

4. Repeat daily until wound has healed.

5. Notify the physician's office if redness or purulent drainage develops. A halo of erythema and a yellow serous quality drainage or fibrinous exudate is normal.

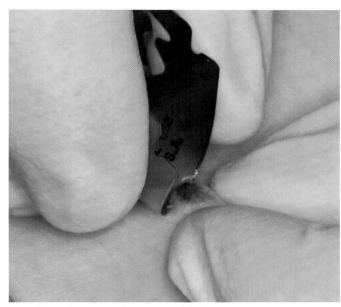

1-3 Shave biopsy with Personna blade.

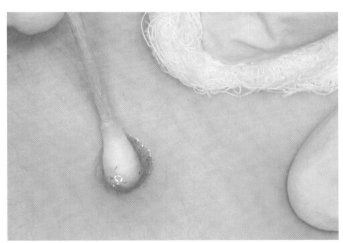

1-4 Application of aluminum chloride solution.

PEARLS/TIPS:

- Although Monsel solution provides better hemostasis, it can tattoo or discolor the skin. Therefore, use aluminum chloride when possible.

- If you suspect a melanoma, excision biopsy may be more appropriate.

- Older or sun-damaged skin heals with less scarring than does younger skin.

- Be sure the lesion is biopsied with adequate depth to permit proper histologic evaluation.

- Lidocaine with epinephrine is **not** used in areas of poor blood supply: fingertips, toes, tip of nose, ear lobes, or penis.

- The smaller the gauge number of the needle, the larger its diameter and the more discomfort it causes the patient.

1b. Punch Biopsy

PURPOSE: Useful for sampling sites of superficial inflammatory and bullous disorders or for benign and malignant skin lesions.

EQUIPMENT NEEDED:

- Sterile instruments: scissors, forceps, needle driver

- Gauze and cotton-tipped swab

- Suture (nylon, plain gut, or Prolene)

- 1% Lidocaine (with epinephrine) for anesthesia

- 3-cc syringe with 22-gauge (or 18-gauge, if preferred) needle to draw up lidocaine

- 30-gauge needle for injection

- Bacitracin ointment (antibacterial)

- Self-adhesive bandage

- Alcohol prep pad or povidone iodine (Betadine) cleanser

- Bottle with tissue preservative

- Disposable cylindrical punch biopsy tool (has a razor-sharp cutting edge)

TECHNIQUE:

1. Swab the area with alcohol prep pad

2. Inject the base of the lesion intradermally with 0.5–1.5 cc of lidocaine with epinephrine. A good

intradermal anesthetic result is a white wheal surrounding the lesion.

3. Stretch the surrounding tissue with thumb and index finger while applying pressure with the punch tool (Figure 1-5).

4. Rotate the punch between the fingers while applying pressure downward. Resistance will cease once you have penetrated the dermis. Cut the plug of tissue deep enough to include subcutaneous tissue.

5. Withdraw the punch and gently elevate the plug of tissue using forceps—take care not to crush the specimen (Figure 1-6). Excise the plug of tissue using sterile scissors.

6. Place the specimen in tissue preservative immediately.

7. Place one or two sutures appropriately to optimize cosmesis (the cosmetic result) and control bleeding (Figure 1-7). The skin should be closed about parallel with existing lines on the skin for the best cosmetic result.

8. Apply a small amount of bacitracin or antibiotic ointment and cover the wound with a self-adhesive bandage.

COMPLICATIONS:

• Transaction of an artery or nerve

POST-PROCEDURE CARE:

Ask patients to follow the instructions listed below for wound care.

1. Keep the original bandage in place for 24 hours, then clean wound once or twice daily with soap and water or hydrogen peroxide.

2. Apply a layer of bacitracin or Polysporin ointment, or petroleum jelly to the area.

3. Cover with self-adhesive bandage (optional).

4. Repeat daily until wound has healed.

5. Notify the physician's office if redness or purulent drainage develops. A halo of erythema and a yellow serous quality drainage or fibrinous exudate is normal.

PEARLS/TIPS:

• In certain anatomic areas, such as the face, important nerves and arteries occur superficially; care must be taken not to transect these structures.

• Biopsies from the scalp and forehead may bleed profusely—be prepared.

• 5.0 or 6.0 suture is best for facial skin.

• 4.0 or 5.0 suture is best for non-facial skin.

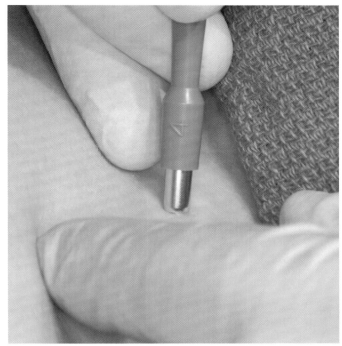

1-5 Punch biopsy.

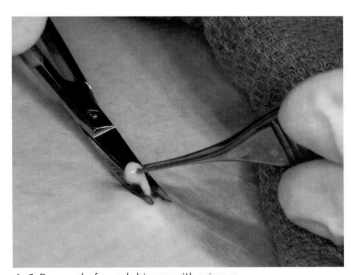

1-6 Removal of punch biopsy with scissors.

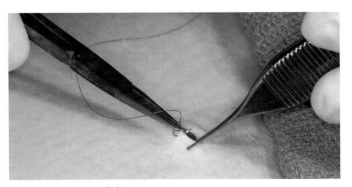

1-7 Suturing punch biopsy.

1c. Elliptical Biopsy or Excision

PURPOSE: Useful for biopsy of deep inflammatory conditions such as panniculitis, or for evaluation of the subcutaneous or fascia layer. Benign and malignant lesions are also sampled or removed in this fashion.

EQUIPMENT NEEDED (FIGURE 1-8):

- Sterile instruments/surgical tray: scissors, forceps, needle driver, scalpel blade (No. 15), skin hook
- Gauze and cotton-tipped swabs
- Suture (nylon, plain gut, or polypropylene) +/− Vicryl (for more detail on suture material, see "2. Suturing")
- 1% Lidocaine (with epinephrine) for anesthesia
- 3-cc syringe with 22-gauge (or 18-gauge if preferred) needle to draw up lidocaine
- 30-gauge needle for injection
- Bacitracin ointment (antibacterial)
- Nonadherent, perforated dressing (e.g., Telfa pad)
- Paper tape
- Alcohol prep
- Antiseptic surgical scrub (e.g., Hibiclens)
- Surgical marking pen
- Bottle with tissue preservative
- Sterile fenestrated drape
- Sterile gloves

TECHNIQUE:

IMPORTANT NOTE: It is prudent to draw out the incision line with a surgical marking pen before anesthesia, because vasoconstriction can obscure the borders of the lesion. Determine proper orientation of the ellipse according to relaxed skin tension lines.

1. Prep the area with Hibiclens or antiseptic surgical scrub.

2. Determine the margins (or amount of normal-appearing tissue you will excise around the lesion). The margins for excising a lesion depend on whether it is a benign or malignant lesion; see Pearls/Tips below for guidelines. The length of a fusiform excision should be three to four times the width to prevent tissue puckering at the elliptical tips when approximating (Figure 1-9).

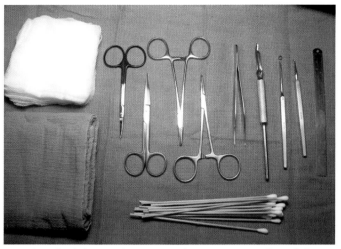

1-8 Standard dermatology surgical tray. Top row (from left to right): gauze, 4-inch curved iris scissors, needle driver, forceps, scalpel, curette, skin hook, and ruler. Bottom row (from left to right): sterile towel, suture scissors, hemostat, and cotton swabs.

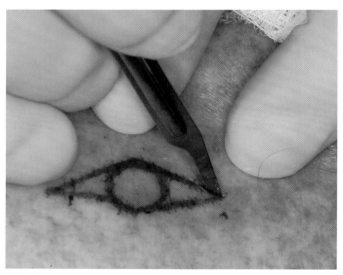

1-9 Markings for fusiform excision.

3. Inject the perilesional skin intradermally and subcutaneously with 1% lidocaine with epinephrine.

4. Incise the skin using a No. 15 scalpel blade, holding the blade handle perpendicular to the skin surface, and draw the blade through the tissue at a 45° angle (Figure 1-9). Minimize the passes through the dermis to reduce "staircasing," which results in ragged edges that are difficult to reapproximate.

5. Hold tension perpendicular to the incision line to stretch the skin as you excise the lesion (Figure 1-10). This will facilitate a smoother glide of the blade through the skin and accentuate the ellipse. The incision should be made at least down to and including subcutaneous tissue, but may include fascia deep to the subcutaneous layer if indicated.

6. Grab the elliptical tip of the tissue gently with forceps or a skin hook and elevate the tissue.

7. Transect the base of the tissue at the desired depth using either the blade or the tissue scissors (Figure 1-11). This is usually at the subcutaneous layer or plane. Be careful to stay in the same plane of tissue as you transect the base of the specimen.

8. Obtain hemostasis by electrocautery or by using stitches to reapproximate the incision.

COMPLICATIONS:

• Bleeding and infection can occur.

POST-PROCEDURE CARE:

Ask patients to follow the instructions listed below for wound care.

1. Keep the original bandage in place for 24 hours, then clean wound once or twice daily with soap and water or hydrogen peroxide.

2. Apply a layer of bacitracin or Polysporin ointment, or petroleum jelly to the area.

3. Cover with self-adhesive bandage (optional).

4. Repeat daily until wound has healed.

5. Notify the physician's office if redness or purulent drainage develops. A halo of erythema and a yellow serous quality drainage or fibrinous exudate is normal.

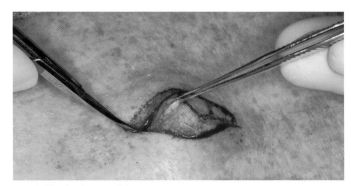

1-10 Beginning excision.

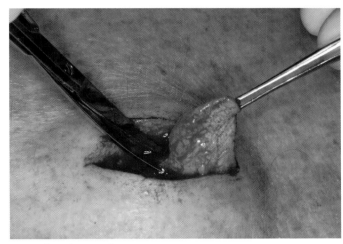

1-11 Base transection.

- For thicker skin, such as that on the back, use a No. 10 scalpel blade.

- For thinner or more delicate areas such as the face, use a No. 15 scalpel blade.

- Be mindful of the underlying anatomy, specifically underlying vessels and nerves.

- When planning your ellipse, pinch the skin in various directions to determine in which axis there will be the least skin tension.

- Consider cosmetic units and try not to cross borders of cosmetic units when planning the ellipse.

- Margins: 1 to 2 mm for benign lesions; 4 mm margins for carcinomas that are a size less than 2 cm; margins for melanoma will depend on depth of invasion.

- Atypical or "dysplastic" nevi may require margins of 4 to 5 mm.

2. Suturing

There are two types of suture material: absorbable and nonabsorbable. The most commonly used nonabsorbable suture for skin procedures are nylon and polypropylene (Prolene). They both cause low to minimal tissue reaction. Commonly used absorbable suture include polyglactin (Vicryl) and surgical gut (plain and chromic).

PURPOSE: Reapproximation of lacerations and surgical wounds.

EQUIPMENT NEEDED (FOR 2A–2F):

- Sterile gloves

- Needle driver

- Forceps

- Skin hook (optional)

- Suture material

- Hydrogen peroxide

- Bacitracin ointment (antibacterial)

- Nonadherent, perforated dressing (e.g., Telfa pad)

- Liquid surgical adhesive (e.g., Mastisol or Benzoin)

- Cotton rolls or folded gauze

- Paper tape or Hypafix dressing retention tape

2a. Instrument Tie

TECHNIQUE:

1. Determine suture size to use on the basis of the anatomic area and wound tension. The wound edges should be easily approximated; therefore, there should not be significant wound tension when placing your top stitches. Deep, absorbable sutures should be placed first if necessary.

2. Grasp your needle driver and place the thumb and ring finger in the loops. The index finger should rest on the hinge while the middle finger flexes to secure the handle. Hold the suture needle between the thumb and index finger and clamp the needle with the needle driver at the base, or swage, of the needle where the suture attaches.

3. Enter the skin perpendicularly with the needle about 2 to 3 mm from the wound edge using a rotary motion with your wrist (Figure 2-1).

4. Stabilize the tissue by gently grasping it with forceps as the needle penetrates the skin. Resistance will be felt until the needle penetrates the dermis.

5. Drive the needle to the appropriate depth at a slightly oblique angle away from the wound edge.

6. Curve the needle across the horizontal plane with a twist or rotation of your wrist. If the wound edges are approximated, you may be able to continue the passage of the needle in a mirror-like fashion into the opposing wound edge with one motion. If the edges are not approximated, you may grasp the emerging needle as it exits the wound edge, at which point you can reposition the needle in the driver and continue the course into the opposing edge. You must be sure that the needle enters the opposing side at the same vertical and horizontal location to prevent tissue override or puckering.

7. Enter the opposing wound edge, advancing the needle horizontally while rotating your wrist. The curve of the needle will direct the tip perpendicular to the dermis.

8. Stabilize the tissue again with your forceps as the needle emerges. The needle should emerge again 2 to 3 mm from the wound edge (Figure 2-2).

9. Prevent backward retraction of the needle as you release the needle driver by grasping the needle tip with your forceps or stabilizing the surrounding tissue with the forceps. Gently grasp the emerging needle with the driver and continue the arc of motion to bring the needle and suture through the tissue.

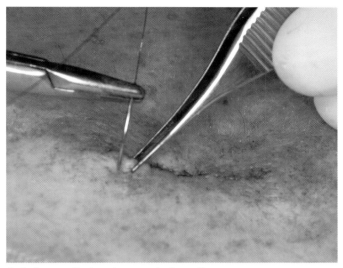

2-1 Perpendicular placement of needle.

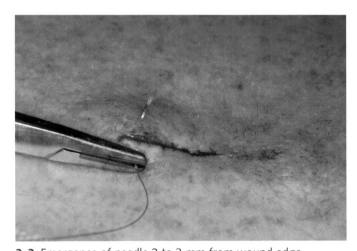

2-2 Emergence of needle 2 to 3 mm from wound edge.

10. Tie a knot. The instrument tie using a surgeon's knot is most common.

   a. Pass the needle through the tissue leaving a short tail of suture.

   b. Hold the suture (needle side of the suture) in your free hand while placing the needle driver between the strand in your hand and the free end of the suture (Figure 2-3).

   c. Wrap the arms of the driver twice with the thread in your hand (Figure 2-4).

   d. Grasp the free end of the suture in the jaws of the driver and bring the knot down flat to the skin surface while crossing your hands, taking care to gently approximate the wound edge (Figure 2-5).

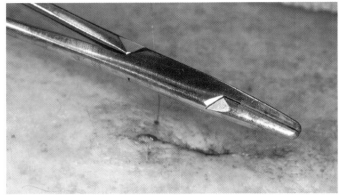

2-3 Initial needle driver placement for instrument tie.

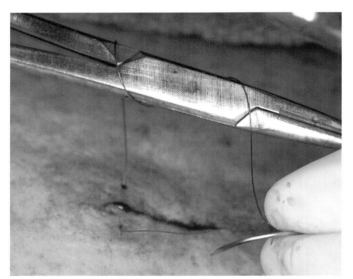

2-4 Suture wrapped twice around needle driver.

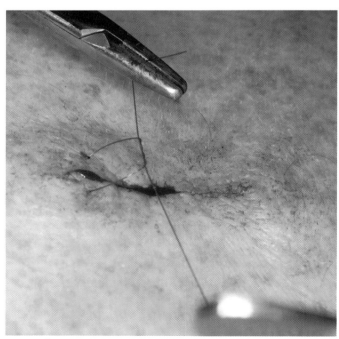

2-5 Pulling suture strands.

e. Do not tighten down the knot too much, because this will strangulate the tissue. The knot should be snug but not tight.

f. Wrap the driver once in the opposite direction for the second throw (Figure 2-6).

g. Tighten the second knot against the first (Figure 2-7). Nylon and polypropylene suture usually require three to five knots to properly secure the suture.

h. Cut the suture 5 to 7 mm above the knot (Figure 2-8).

2b. Buried Suture

Buried sutures are used to close dead space and approximate the wound edges. This will minimize tension on the surface stitches and allow removal of the top suture sooner to prevent "railroad tracking" and/or wound dehiscence. Before placing your suture (according to technique described in "2a. Instrument Tie"), it may be necessary to excise the wound edge to allow for better eversion of the wound edge and to minimize wound tension and maximize cosmesis. This can be done in the subcutaneous plane using blunt or sharp dissection. If necessary, the subcutaneous plane can be approximated using absorbable suture material. Because the subcutaneous tissue lacks connective tissue, it is necessary to take generous bites of tissue, or the suture will easily tear through.

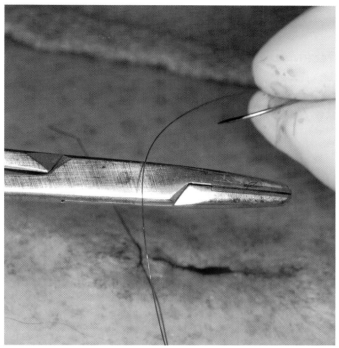

2-6 Suture wrapped once around needle driver in opposite direction.

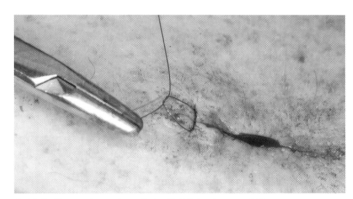

2-7 Pulling suture strands to finish instrument tie.

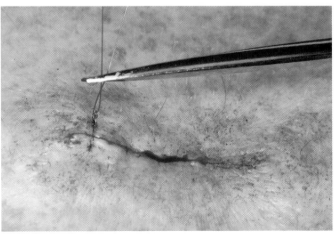

2-8 Cutting suture.

2c. Dermal Buried Suture

TECHNIQUE:

1. Use Vicryl or another absorbable suture.

2. Pass the needle into the deep side of one edge of the wound (Figure 2-9).

3. Advance the needle obliquely toward the wound edge to exit just below the epidermis (Figure 2-10). If the needle exits too high, it will cause inversion of the wound edge, resulting in more scarring. If it exits too deep, it will not attain meticulous approximation of the epidermis.

4. Reposition the needle in the driver and enter the opposing edge superficially just below the epidermis.

5. Advance the needle obliquely downward and with a rotation of the wrist, and arc the needle tip back toward the wound edge (Figure 2-11).

6. Cut the suture just above the knot to leave the least amount of suture, to minimize suture reaction or spitting (Figure 2-12). Vicryl suture needs three knots per stitch to stay in place.

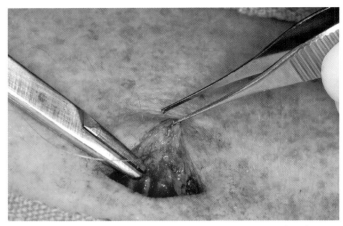

2-9 Absorbable suture is passed through the deep side of wound edge.

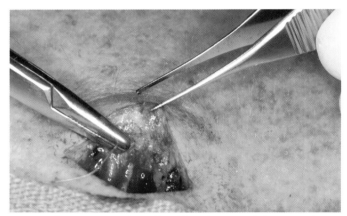

2-10 Advancement of needle obliquely toward the wound edge to exit just below the epidermis.

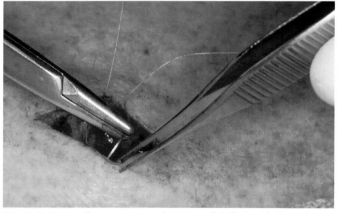

2-11 Entering the opposing edge superficially just below the epidermis.

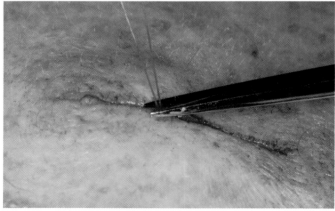

2-12 Suture is cut just above the knot.

2d. Running Suture Versus Interrupted Suture

The advantages of a running suture are that it saves time and conserves suture. The wound should be approximated with dermal suture or be under minimal tension. Nonabsorbable suture is generally used. The risk of dehiscence is greater if the suture breaks. Interrupted sutures offer the advantage of wound security but are much more time consuming and you will use more suture.

TECHNIQUE:

1. Tie a knot at the end of the incision to begin. The end of the suture attached to the needle is left uncut.

2. Place continuous loops down the incision line (Figure 2-13).

3. Tie a final knot at the end of the incision line. Since you only have one working suture strand (which is attached to the needle), a second strand can be created by using the loop from the last throw as one of the ends. The loop will need to be long enough to create enough knots to secure the suture in place (Figure 2-14).

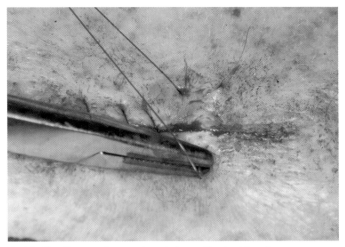

2-13 Continuous loops placed down the incision line.

2e. Staples

Staples can be used to close a wound instead of sutures, and offer the advantage of low tissue reaction, good strength, and time reduction. They are designed to provide good wound eversion and create less tissue damage. They are most often used on the trunk, extremities, and scalp. Removal is simple with the appropriate staple removal devices that are available. However, staples are more costly than suture and are not as useful on the face, where meticulous approximation is necessary to maximize cosmesis.

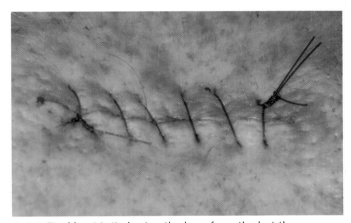

2-14 Final knot is tied using the loop from the last throw.

EQUIPMENT NEEDED:

- Sterile staple device
- Two forceps

TECHNIQUE:

1. Evert the wound edges gently with the two forceps by grasping and turning the edges outward so that the dermis is exposed. It is important to gently evert the wound edges before staple placement.

2. Have another individual then place the staples, using the staple device.

3. Place a staple approximately every centimeter (1 cm apart) until the wound is closed.

2f. Two-Handed Surgical Tie (Square Knot)

TECHNIQUE:

1. Place one suture strand between index finger and thumb of each hand (Figure 2-15).

2. Place strand from left hand between right thumb and index finger (Figure 2-16).

3. Close right thumb and index finger so that both strands are cradled in the opening created by your thumb and index finger (Figure 2-17).

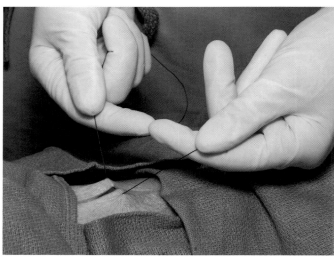

2-15 Place both suture strands between index finger and thumb of both hands.

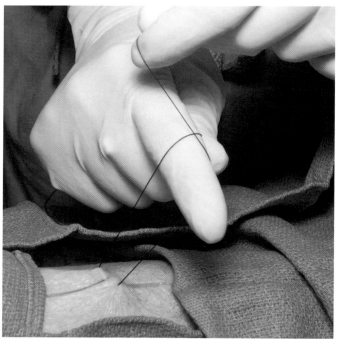

2-16 Place strand from left hand between right thumb and index finger.

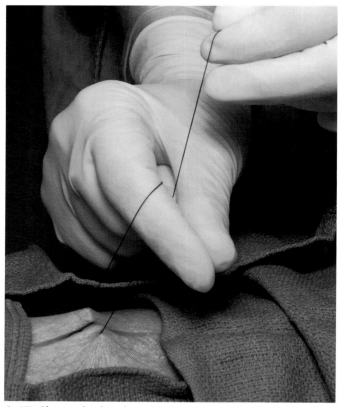

2-17 Close right thumb and index finger so that both strands are cradled in the opening created by your thumb and index finger.

4. Turn right hand outward in a pronating motion, pushing the thumb and index finger through the loop (Figures 2-18a and 2-18b).

5. Place strand from left hand between right index finger and thumb (Figure 2-19).

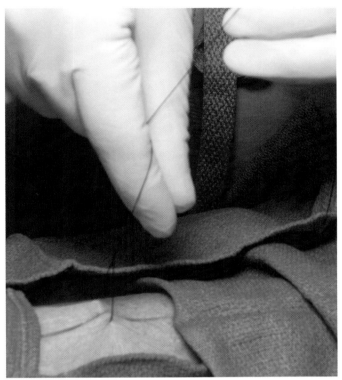

2-18a Turn right hand outward in a pronating motion, pushing the thumb and index finger through the loop.

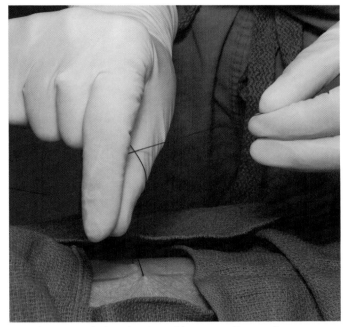

2-18b Turn right hand outward in a pronating motion, pushing the thumb and index finger through the loop.

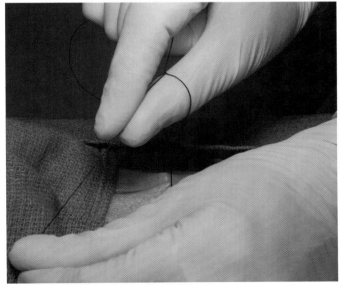

2-19 Place strand from left hand between right index finger and thumb.

6. Turn right hand inward in a supinating motion, while still grasping the strand, pushing the thumb and index finger through the loop (Figures 2-20a and 2-20b).

7. Pull remaining strand through the loop (Figure 2-21).

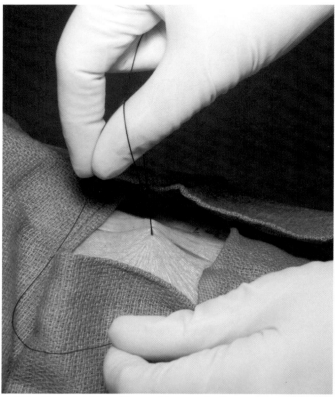

2-20a Turn right hand inward in a supinating motion while still grasping the strand, pushing the thumb and index finger through the loop.

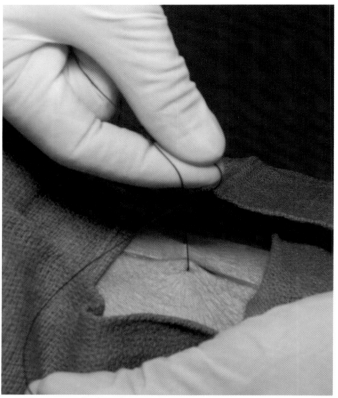

2-20b Turn right hand inward in a supinating motion while still grasping the strand, pushing the thumb and index finger through the loop.

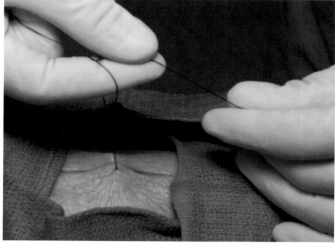

2-21 Pull remaining strand through the loop.

Optional: For a double throw, repeat steps 4 through 7 (Figures 2-22a and 2-22b).

8. Pull both strands in horizontal motion with equal tension, carefully aligning wound edges (Figure 2-23).

9. Place right strand over right thumb (Figure 2-24),

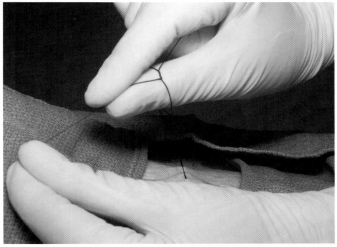

2-22a Optional: For a double throw, repeat steps 4 through 7.

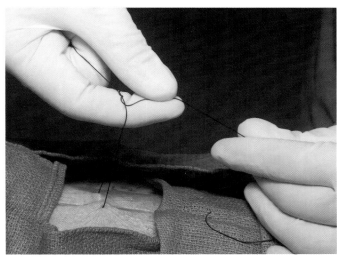

2-22b Optional: For a double throw, repeat steps 4 through 7.

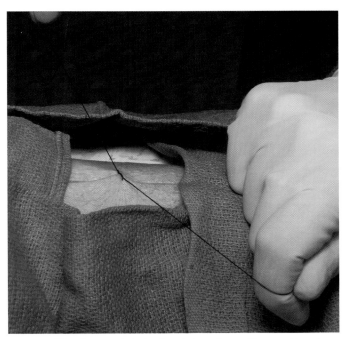

2-23 Pull both strands in horizontal motion with equal tension, carefully aligning wound edges.

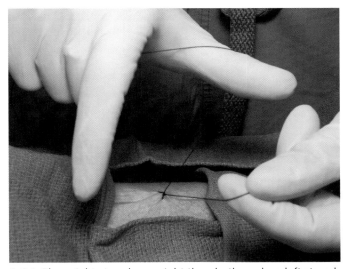

2-24 Place right strand over right thumb, then place left strand between right thumb and index finger.

then place left strand between right thumb and index finger (Figure 2-25).

10. Close right thumb and index finger so that both strands are cradled in the opening created by your thumb and index finger (Figure 2-26).

11. Turn right hand inward in a supinating motion, pushing the index finger and thumb through the loop (Figure 2-27).

12. Place strand from left hand between the right index finger and thumb (Figure 2-28).

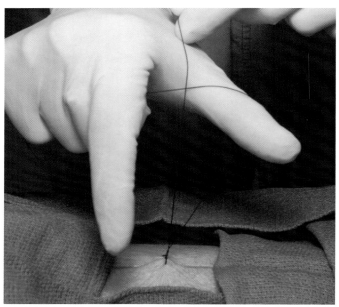

2-25 Place right strand over right thumb, then place left strand between right thumb and index finger.

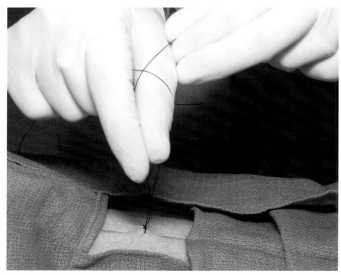

2-26 Close right thumb and index finger so that both strands are cradled in the opening created by your thumb and index finger.

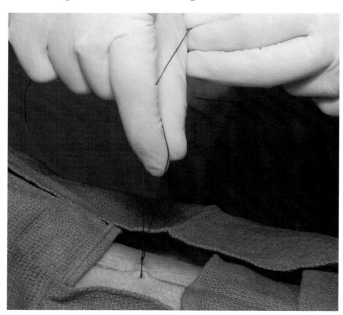

2-27 Turn right hand inward in a supinating motion, pushing the index finger and thumb through the loop.

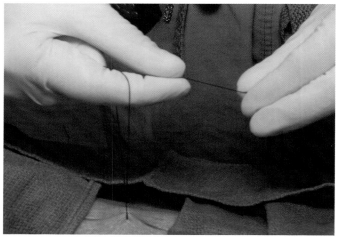

2-28 Place strand from left hand between the right index finger and thumb.

13. Turn right hand outward in a pronating motion, while grasping the strand, pushing the thumb and index finger through the loop (Figure 2-29).

14. Pull remaining strand through the loop (Figure 2-30).

15. Pull both strands in horizontal motion with equal tension, finishing the knot (Figure 2-31).

COMPLICATIONS (FOR 2A–2F):

- Bleeding/hematoma
- Infection
- Nerve damage
- Scarring
- Pain
- Allergic contact dermatitis to tape, adhesive, or antibiotic ointment
- Wound dehiscence

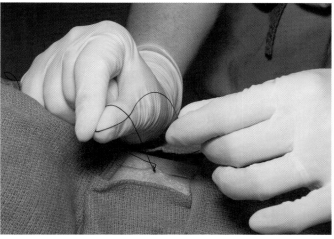

2-29 Turn right hand outward in a pronating motion while grasping the strand, pushing the thumb and index finger through the loop.

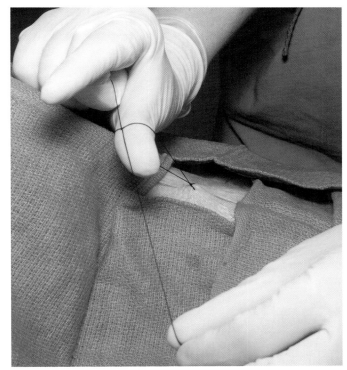

2-30 Pull remaining strand through the loop.

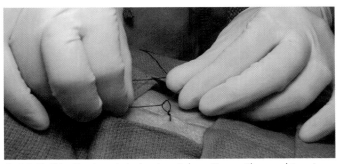

2-31 Pull both strands in horizontal motion with equal tension, finishing the knot.

POST-PROCEDURE CARE (FOR 2A-2F):

Surgical wounds should be dressed in the following manner:

1. Clean the incision line with peroxide.

2. Apply bacitracin ointment to the wound (Figure 2-32).

3. Cut a Telfa pad to fit over the suture line (Figure 2-33).

4. Place cotton rolls or folded gauze over the Telfa pad (Figure 2-34).

5. Apply a liquid surgical adhesive such as Mastisol or Benzoin (Figure 2-35).

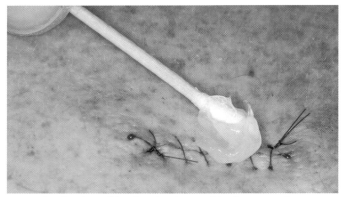

2-32 Application of bacitracin ointment to the wound.

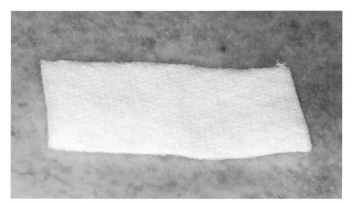

2-33 Placement of Telfa pad.

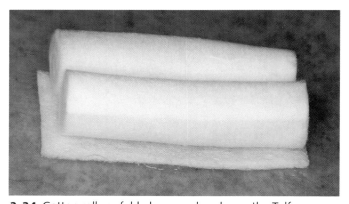

2-34 Cotton rolls or folded gauze placed over the Telfa.

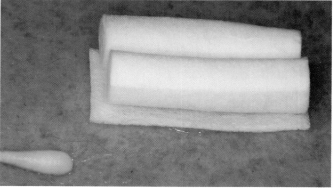

2-35 Application of adhesive.

6. Make a pressure bandage by taping the dressing in place with paper tape or, preferably, Hypafix (Figures 2-36a and 2-36b).

7. Leave the dressing in place for 24 to 48 hours.

8. Use 1/2 peroxide and water to clean off any scab or serous debris after the initial bandage is removed, then apply bacitracin or petroleum jelly and a light bandage.

PEARLS/TIPS (for 2a–2f):

- Prolene suture is much easier to remove, but requires meticulous knot tying because the knots do not hold as well.

- Leave facial sutures in for 5 to 7 days.

- Leave sutures in the extremities and trunk in for 9 to 12 days.

- It may be necessary to leave sutures in extensor surfaces and the thin skin of the groin for up to 2 weeks.

- The longer sutures remain, the more difficult it is to remove them and the more likely "railroad tracking" is; however, you must leave sutures in long enough to prevent dehiscence.

- Whenever possible, use lidocaine with epinephrine to minimize bleeding.

- Scalp and facial incisions tend to bleed profusely.

- Use preoperative antibiotics in susceptible patients (such as those with artificial valves or joints).

- If you get a difficult "bleeder," don't panic. Apply firm, direct, uninterrupted pressure for 5 to 15 minutes to allow clotting to take place.

- A proper pressure bandage is critical to prevent postoperative bleeding. Ensure that the patient is positioned in a manner that minimizes wound tension while the bandage is applied so that when he or she relaxes, the bandage applies proper pressure. For example, for vertical incisions on the upper back, make sure the shoulders are rolled back (tell the patient to touch the shoulder blades together) while you bandage. When the shoulders relax, the bandage will be brought more firmly against the wound. The tightness of the bandage will remind the patient not to roll the shoulders forward to the point that the sutures are under too much tension.

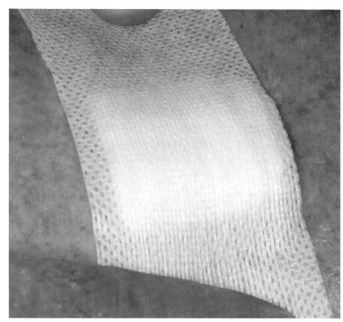

2-36a Pressure bandage placement with Hypafix.

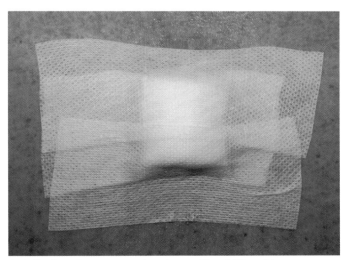

2-36b Securing pressure bandage with additional tape.

3. Cyst Removal

PURPOSE: Several techniques exist for the removal of epidermal cysts. Although incision and drainage of a cyst with subsequent expression of the cyst wall can occasionally be performed, excision of the cyst with careful dissection of the cyst wall from the surrounding skin is usually necessary to prevent recurrence. In general, it is prudent not to treat a cyst that is actively infected or inflamed, because this will increase the risk of postoperative infection or other complications.

EQUIPMENT NEEDED:

- No. 15 scalpel blade
- Hibiclens or antiseptic surgical scrub
- Surgical marking pen
- 1% Lidocaine (with epinephrine) for anesthesia
- Choose suture appropriate for anatomical area (e.g., absorbent suture for subcutaneous closure)

TECHNIQUE:

1. Cleanse the area with Hibiclens or antiseptic surgical scrub.

2. Mark the borders of the cyst with a surgical marking pen before injecting anesthesia, otherwise the fluid will obscure the borders of the cyst (Figure 3-1).

3. Anesthetize the surrounding and overlying tissue with 1% lidocaine with epinephrine (Figure 3-2). It may be difficult to anesthetize the base of the cyst initially if the cyst is very large; however, this can be done later once the cyst is partly removed and the base is more visible.

4. Examine epidermal inclusion cysts for a central punctum or drainage point, which is a site of potential recurrence. This point should be marked and excised with the cyst.

5. Use a No. 15 scalpel blade to make a linear or small elliptical incision over the surface of the cyst (Figure 3-3). The amount of skin excised should circumscribe only a small portion of the cyst surface area (Figure 3-4).

6. Carry the incision down to the level of the glistening cyst wall, but do not rupture the cyst.

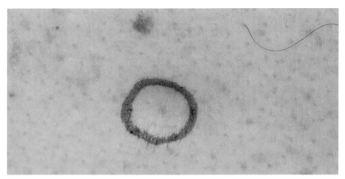

3-1 Mark the borders of the cyst with a surgical marking pen prior to injection of anesthesia as the fluid will obscure the borders of the cyst.

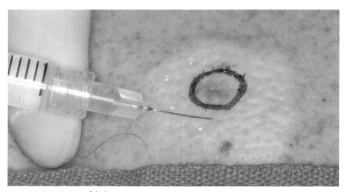

3-2 Injection of lidocaine.

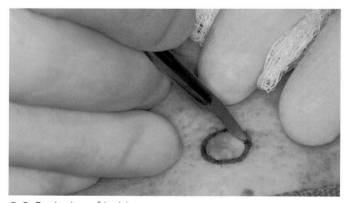

3-3 Beginning of incision.

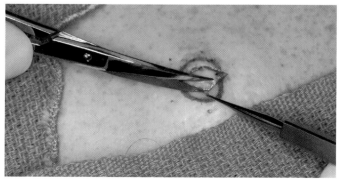

3-4 Separation of cyst wall from surrounding tissue.

7. Elevate the lateral skin edge and carefully dissect the cyst wall from the surrounding tissue using blunt and/or sharp dissection with your scissors (Figure 3-5).

8. Elevate the cyst and visualize its base as you free the lateral cyst wall. At this point, it may be necessary to inject additional anesthesia at the base (Figure 3-6).

9. Try to excise the entire cyst without rupturing the wall; however, if you happen to leave a portion of the cyst wall behind, it will be necessary to remove these remaining fragments to prevent recurrence.

10. Watch cysts that have ruptured in the past and left scar tissue with sinus tracking. These sinus tracks will also need excision, or recurrence is likely.

11. Use a layered closure, if necessary, to close the dead space created by the removal of the cyst. Underlying subcutaneous tissue should be approximated with absorbable suture before placement of your top stitches (Figure 3-7).

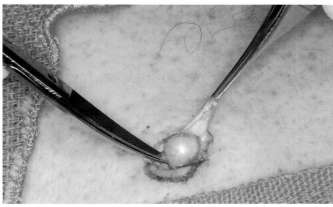

3-5 Elevation of the lateral skin edge and dissection of the cyst wall from the surrounding tissue using blunt and/or sharp dissection with scissors.

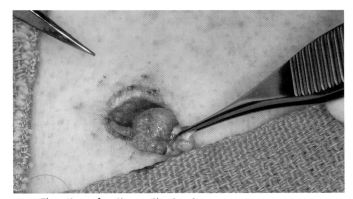

3-6 Elevation of entire cystic structure.

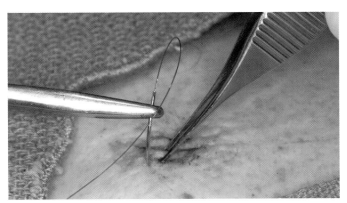

3-7 Placement of top stitches.

COMPLICATIONS:

- Bleeding

- Infection

- Cyst reoccurrence if the entire cyst wall was not removed

POST-PROCEDURE CARE:

Ask patients to follow the instructions listed below for wound care.

1. Keep the original bandage in place for 24 hours, then clean wound once or twice daily with soap and water or hydrogen peroxide.

2. Apply a layer of bacitracin or bacitracin-polymyxin B (Polysporin) ointment, or petroleum jelly to the area.

3. Cover with self-adhesive bandage (optional).

4. Repeat daily until wound has healed.

5. Notify the physician's office if redness or purulent drainage develops. A halo of erythema and a yellow serous quality drainage or fibrinous exudate is normal.

PEARLS/TIPS:

- Every attempt possible should be made to remove the cyst while it is completely intact, to avoid cyst reoccurence.

4. Incision and Drainage of Abscesses

PURPOSE: The primary management of abscesses, furuncles, and infected cysts should be incision and drainage (I&D). Culture of purulent material may be indicated in some instances but is usually not necessary. The appropriate time for I&D of a lesion is when the overlying skin has become thinned and soft, which indicates that the lesion has cavitated. Using warm compresses for 24 to 48 hours before the procedure can help soften the lesion and facilitate I&D.

EQUIPMENT NEEDED:

- No. 11 scalpel blade

- 1% Lidocaine with epinephrine for anesthesia

- 1/4 inch iodoform gauze

- Cotton-tipped swab or curette

- Sterile 4 inch x 4 inch gauze

- Protective shielding (mask with face shield, or mask and protective eyewear)

TECHNIQUE:

1. Anesthetize the surrounding and overlying skin with 1% lidocaine with epinephrine. You will notice that it will be more difficult to completely numb the area because of the intense inflammation.

2. Insert a No. 11 scalpel blade into the center of the lesion in a cross-hatch pattern.

3. Watch for explosive expression of purulent material as the blade enters the lesion. It is prudent to cover the area with gauze or use protective shielding while inserting the blade.

4. Press the surrounding tissue gently to express as much material as possible. Because abscesses are often loculated, you will need to insert a cotton-tipped swab or curette into the cavity and break up the adhesions or loculations to promote the removal of as much purulent material as possible.

5. Place a ribbon of 1/4-inch iodoform gauze into the cavity once the abscess is decompressed, taking care not to over-pack the wound; place enough gauze into the wound to wick out any serous or purulent drainage that may reaccumulate. Try to place the gauze in pleats to loosely pack the wound. This will also keep the incision site patent until the cavity has healed from the inside out.

6. Bandage the wound with 4 inch $\times$ 4 inch gauze to absorb the drainage. The frequency of dressing changes and application of 1/4-inch packing gauze will depend on the amount of drainage from the wound, but should be done at least once a day. Each day, less packing material will be needed as the wound continues to heal.

7. Place the patient on the appropriate antibiotics.

COMPLICATIONS:

- Bleeding

- Infection does not improve

POST-PROCEDURE CARE:

1. Continue at least daily repacking of wound until healed.

2. Instruct patient to notify the physician's office if wound does not appear to be healing, erythema spreads, severe pain develops at wound site, or a fever develops.

3. Instruct patient to take all antibiotics prescribed, even if the wound appears to be improving.

- Patient education is the key to the success of the wound healing process. Make certain that the patient and at least one member of the family (if possible) understands how to change the packing material and dress the wound properly. Also emphasize the importance of changing the packing at least once a day.

5. Removal of Ingrown Nail

PURPOSE: To remove an ingrown nail.

EQUIPMENT NEEDED (FIGURE 5-1):

- Routine surgical tray
- Freer elevator
- Anvil action nail splitter
- Nail pulling forceps
- 1% Lidocaine without epinephrine for nerve block
- Antiseptic surgical scrub (e.g., Hibiclens)
- Tourniquet
- No. 2 or 3 curette
- 4.0 polypropylene (Prolene) suture
- Hemostatic agent (gel foam)
- Bacitracin
- Nonadherent, perforated dressing (e.g., Telfa pad)
- Rolled gauze
- Hypafix dressing retention tape
- Coban self-adherent wrap
- Liquid surgical adhesive (e.g., Mastisol)
- 22- or 18-gauge needle to draw up lidocaine
- 30-gauge needle for injection

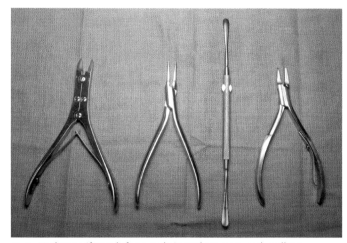

5-1 Nail tray (from left to right): nail nipper, nail-pulling forceps, freer elevator, and anvil action nail splitter.

TECHNIQUE:

IMPORTANT NOTE: A digital block can be performed using 1% lidocaine *without* epinephrine. It is best to perform the nerve block 15 to 20 minutes before the procedure (although good anesthetic effect can occur within 5 to 10 minutes). Inject 1 cc of the lidocaine into each side of the base of the digit (medial and lateral). Infiltrate the subcutaneous layer in a radial fashion to include the dorsal and ventral portion of the digit. This will require a total of 2–4 cc of the lidocaine.

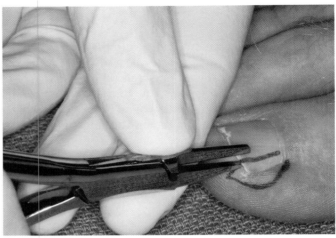

5-2 Removal of nail plate using nail splitter.

1. Cleanse the affected digit with Hibiclens.

2. Wait 15 to 20 minutes for the nerve block. (Refer to Important Note above.)

3. Inject 1% lidocaine without epinephrine into the proximal and lateral nail folds and, finally, into the tip of the digit.

4. Apply a tourniquet for a short period of time, using hemostats to clamp the tourniquet during the procedure to control bleeding.

5. Use the nail splitter to split away a 3- to 4-mm portion of the nail plate on the involved side (Figure 5-2). Removal of the entire nail plate is usually not necessary.

6. Insert the freer elevator under the nail plate and slide the instrument under the entire longitudinal length of the nail to detach the nail plate from the nail bed.

7. Use the freer elevator to detach the nail plate from the proximal nail fold. Grab the nail plate with hemostats or nail forceps and gently extract the freed nail with a pulling and twisting motion. This will expose the nail bed, matrix, and lateral fold.

8. Check whether the lateral fold has become inflamed and hypertrophic. Elliptical excision of this overriding skin is performed (Figure 5-3).

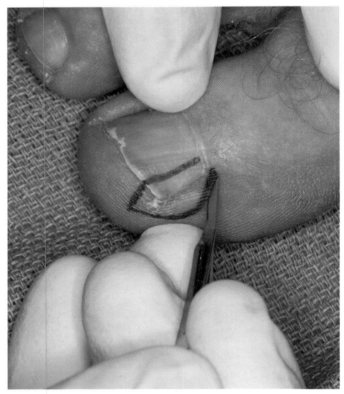

5-3 Elliptical excision of this overriding skin.

9. Follow this with light electrocautery to control bleeding.

10. Make an oblique incision at the juncture of the proximal and lateral nail fold to expose the proximal nail matrix.

11. Partial matricectomy is done easily by electrodesiccation and curettage. This also facilitates hemostasis.

   a. Use a No. 2 or 3 curette to vigorously curette the nail matrix, and follow with electrodesiccation. Make 2 or 3 passes with this technique.

   b. Use 4.0 polypropylene to suture the oblique incision that was made to expose the proximal nail matrix.

12. Place a hemostatic agent into the excised portion of the lateral nail fold.

COMPLICATIONS:

- Bleeding

- Infection does not improve

POST-PROCEDURE CARE:

1. Pack the excised portion of the nail fold with hemostatic agent.

2. Apply layer of bacitracin.

3. Apply a Telfa pad.

4. Use tightly rolled gauze or dental rolls as next layer.

5. Apply liquid surgical adhesive to exposed peripheral skin.

6. Tape the bandage material into place with longitudinal orientation of Hypafix (do not apply Hypafix circumferentially). Coban wrap can then be used circumferentially if additional pressure is necessary, taking care not to constrict the blood supply.

PEARLS/TIPS:

- Postoperative pain is common and may be significant.

- Keep off the foot for 24 hours and keep elevated when possible.

- Ingrown nails are commonly colonized or overtly infected; it is better to treat "infected" nails with antibiotics before surgical intervention.

III. Head and Neck

6. Ear Wax (Cerumen) Removal

PURPOSE: To improve hearing.

EQUIPMENT NEEDED (FIGURE 6-1):

- Ear loop/curette
- Plastic basin
- Warm water and hydrogen peroxide
- Syringe (usually made of metal) with at least 30 cc capacity, or a specially designed bottle with tubing attached (Figure 6-1)
- Otoscope

TECHNIQUE #1—EAR LOOP/CURETTE:

1. Inspect the patient's ears with the otoscope.
2. Push the glass window of the otoscope aside and, with direct visualization, insert the ear loop through the window.
3. Remove the cerumen using a scooping motion toward you.

TECHNIQUE #2—IRRIGATION:

1. Inspect the patient's ears with an otoscope.
2. Fill a plastic basin with a 1:1 ratio mixture of warm water and hydrogen peroxide (the hydrogen peroxide will soften the cerumen).
3. Place a towel on the patient's shoulder and place the basin just below the ear.
4. Fill the syringe with water and hydrogen peroxide mixture.
5. Place the tip of the syringe gently to just within the first part of the external ear canal (Figure 6-2).
6. Push on the plunger of the syringe and flush the water-hydrogen peroxide into the ear canal, directing the tip of the syringe toward the occiput and superiorly—do not place it toward the tympanic membrane. The pressure of the water will cause small pieces of cerumen to come out; flush until cleared.

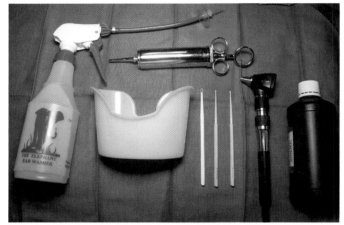

6-1 Equipment for ear wax removal (from left to right): spray bottle with attachment, metal syringe, plastic basin, three ear loops, otoscope, and hydrogen peroxide.

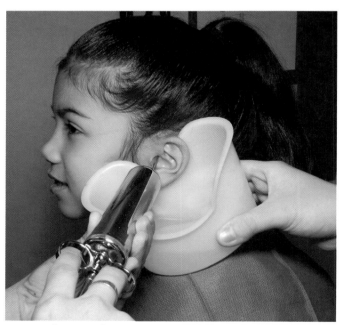

6-2 Application of pressured water into ear canal via metal syringe.

COMPLICATIONS:

- Nausea, nystagmus (usually occurs if the water is too cold)
- Flushing water into the ear canal may stimulate the cough reflex in rare cases
- Inability to remove all of the wax

POST-PROCEDURE CARE:

1. Inspect the ear canal with the otoscope. If the external canal is inflamed, consider a prescription to treat otitis externa; inspect the tympanic membrane for perforations.

2. No formal follow up is required, but this is a recurring condition in adults and you will want to check the patient's ears regularly during follow-up visits.

PEARLS/TIPS:

- If the cerumen is difficult to remove, give the patient a prescription for an earwax softener.

7. Removal of a Foreign Body from the Eye: Conjunctival

PURPOSE: To remove a foreign object, improve vision, or decrease the chance of conjunctival infection or damage.

EQUIPMENT NEEDED (FIGURE 7-1):

- Eye chart for distant and near vision
- Penlight
- Topical ophthalmoplegic anesthetic
- Fluorescein ophthalmic staining strips
- Cobalt blue light source (Wood's lamp or cobalt blue penlight)
- Magnifying glasses (attached to a headset)
- Sterile normal saline for irrigation
- Cotton-tipped applicators (premoistened with saline)
- 18-gauge needle with a small syringe

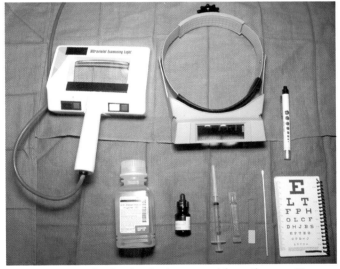

7-1 Equipment for foreign body removal from the eye. Top row (from left to right): cobalt blue light source, magnifying glass attached to a headset. Bottom row (from left to right): sterile saline, topical ophthalmoplegic anesthetic, 18-gauge needle with a small syringe, sterile saline in a dropper applicator, fluorescein, cotton-tipped applicator, and eye chart.

TECHNIQUE:

1. Document visual acuity before beginning the procedure using the eye chart.

2. Instill one drop of the anesthetic agent in the affected eye and have the patient blink a few times. Warn the patient that he or she may experience a stinging or burning sensation.

3. Inspect the conjunctiva once the stinging or burning sensation subsides. Have the patient look up, down, and toward both the nasal and temporal sides. Evert both the upper and lower eyelids and inspect the mucosa.

4. Stain the eye with fluorescein by placing the strip inside the lower eyelid and having the patient blink their eye several times to spread the dye (Figures 7-2a and 7-2b).

5. Place the headset with the magnifying lenses around your forehead. Keep the cobalt blue light source ready.

6. Turn off the lights and inspect the conjunctiva using the cobalt blue light source. Have the patient look up, down, and toward both the nasal and temporal sides. Evert both the upper and lower eyelids and inspect the mucosa (Figure 7-3). **Fluorescein binds to corneal stroma and devitalized epithelium; therefore, the area that is damaged will fluoresce when highlighted with the cobalt blue light source.**

7. Use the premoistened cotton-tipped applicator to gently remove the foreign body.

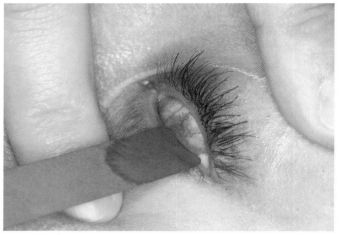

7-2a Application of fluorescein to eye.

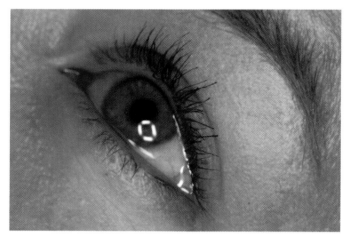

7-2b After fluorescein application.

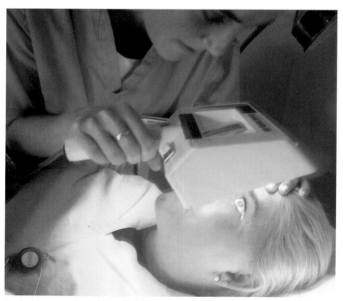

7-3 Using cobalt blue light source to identify foreign body in eye.

8. Irrigate the eye with at least 100 cc of sterile normal saline to remove the fluorescein dye (Figure 7-4).

COMPLICATIONS:

- Incomplete removal of the foreign body

- Infection

- Scarring

- Permanent visual impairment

POST-PROCEDURE CARE:

1. Patching the eye is controversial, but many physicians continue to do so.

2. Make sure that the patient has adequate pain medication, and have the patient follow up in 24 hours for an eye re-examination to ensure that healing has occurred.

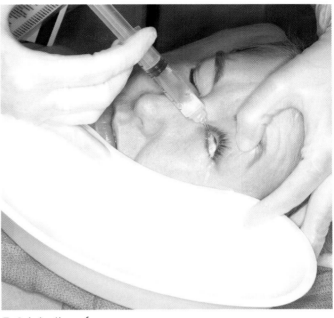

7-4 Irrigation of eye.

PEARLS/TIPS:

- While performing the procedure, it is helpful to ask the patient to focus on one spot and not to move their eyes.

- You should also attempt to calm the patient by distracting with conversation while you perform the procedure.

8. Removal of a Foreign Body from the Eye: Corneal

PURPOSE: To remove a foreign object, improve vision, or decrease the chance for corneal infection or damage.

EQUIPMENT NEEDED (SEE FIGURE 7-1):

- Eye chart for distant and near vision

- Penlight

- Topical ophthalmoplegic anesthetic

- Fluorescein ophthalmic staining strips

- Cobalt blue light source (Wood's lamp or cobalt blue penlight)

- Magnifying glasses (attached to a headset)

- Sterile normal saline for irrigation

- Cotton-tipped applicators (premoistened with saline)

- 18-gauge needle with a small syringe

TECHNIQUE:

1. Document visual acuity before beginning the procedure using the eye chart.

2. Instill one drop of the anesthetic agent in the affected eye and have the patient blink a few times. Warn the patient that he or she may experience a stinging or burning sensation.

3. Inspect the conjunctiva and cornea once the stinging or burning sensation subsides. Have the patient look up, down, and toward both the nasal and temporal sides. Evert both the upper and lower eyelids and inspect the mucosa.

4. Use a premoistened cotton-tipped applicator to remove any visible foreign bodies.

5. Stain the eye with fluorescein by placing the strip inside the lower eyelid and having the patient blink their eye several times to spread the dye (see Figures 7-2a and 7-2b).

6. Place the headset with the magnifying lenses around your forehead. Keep the cobalt blue light source ready.

7. Turn off the lights and inspect the cornea using the cobalt blue light source. Have the patient look up, down, and toward both the nasal and temporal sides. Evert both the upper and lower eyelids and inspect the mucosa (see Figure 7-3). **Fluorescein binds to corneal stroma and devitalized epithelium; therefore, the area that is damaged will fluoresce when highlighted with the cobalt blue light source.**

8. Use a sterile 18-gauge needle to approach the foreign body at a tangential angle to the eyeball with the needle bevel upwards. Hold the syringe using a pencil grip for improved control. Lift the object gently from its bed with the needle tip. If a residual corneal rust ring is present, it can occasionally be removed with the sterile needle.

9. Irrigate the eye with at least 100 cc of sterile normal saline to remove the fluorescein dye.

COMPLICATIONS:

- Incomplete removal of the foreign body
- Infection
- Scarring
- Permanent visual impairment
- Perforation of the cornea or globe

POST-PROCEDURE CARE:

1. Patching the eye is controversial, but many physicians continue to do so.

2. Make sure that the patient has adequate pain medication, and have the patient follow up in 24 hours for eye re-examination to ensure that healing has occurred.

PEARLS/TIPS:

- While performing the procedure, it is helpful to ask the patient to focus on one spot and not to move their eyes.

- You should also attempt to calm the patient by distracting with conversation while you perform the procedure.

9. Removal of a Foreign Body from the Ear

PURPOSE: To remove a foreign body from the external auditory canal.

EQUIPMENT NEEDED (FIGURE 9-1):

- Otoscope

- Blunt-tipped, right-angled Day hook, small wire loop curette, Hartman forceps, or alligator forceps

- Irrigation solution

- Suction

- Papoose board (for restraint if necessary)

TECHNIQUE:

1. Have the patient positioned and still.

2. Use the otoscope to visually examine the canal. This exam is important not only to locate the foreign body, but also to inspect the canal for abrasions, lacerations, or perforation of the tympanic membrane.

3. Look carefully for objects embedded in cerumen, and remove cerumen using a loop as needed.

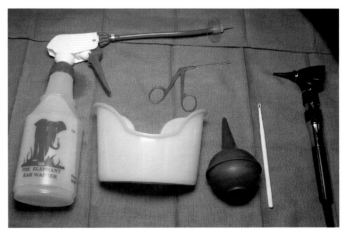

9-1 Equipment for foreign body removal from ear (from left to right): spray bottle with attachment, plastic basin, alligator forceps, suction bulb, loop curette, and otoscope.

4. Use the above-mentioned instruments to carefully remove the object (Figure 9-2). Spherical objects are best removed using the Day hook or suction.

COMPLICATIONS:

- Mucosal injury during attempted removal
- Perforation of the tympanic membrane

POST-PROCEDURE CARE:

1. Perform a visual examination of the canal for mucosal injury and tympanic membrane perforation.

PEARLS/TIPS:

- If the object is not readily removed or the patient is uncooperative, refer to an otolaryngologist for removal.
- In patients with traumatic perforation, there is the possibility of middle or inner ear damage, and an otolaryngologist should see these patients.
- Symptoms of hearing loss, vertigo, or nystagmus indicate the need for urgent otolaryngologic consultation.
- Foreign objects in the ear may result in purulent, foul-smelling discharge.

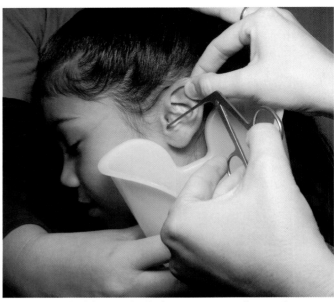

9-2 Removal of foreign body from ear using alligator forceps.

10. Removal of a Foreign Body from the Nose

PURPOSE: To remove a foreign body from the nasal canal.

EQUIPMENT NEEDED (FIGURE 10-1):

- Adequate light source
- Nasal speculum
- Hartman forceps, small wire loop curette, right-angle Day hook, or alligator forceps
- Topical anesthetic spray (optional)
- Topical vasoconstrictor (optional)
- Papoose board (for restraint if necessary)
- Suction and swabs

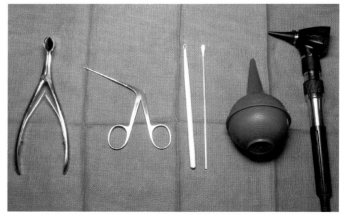

10-1 Equipment for foreign body removal from nose (from left to right): nasal speculum, alligator forceps, loop curette, cotton-tipped applicator, suction bulb, and otoscope (used as light source).

TECHNIQUE:

1. Apply topical medications if applicable.

2. Arrange the patient so they are supine with their head tilted back.

3. Introduce the nasal speculum into the nare.

4. Position the speculum so that it will open vertically. Putting pressure on the nasal septum is quite painful.

5. Remove discharge with suction or a swab. With objects anterior to the nasal turbinates, removal may be attempted by suction or with the instruments listed above (Figure 10-2).

COMPLICATIONS:

• Mucosal injury resulting from trauma during attempted removal

• Aspiration or laryngeal obstruction if the foreign body is dislodged into the nasopharynx

POST-PROCEDURE CARE:

1. Inspect for mucosal injury and respiratory status.

PEARLS/TIPS:

• A foreign body in the nose will often result in unilateral purulent, foul-smelling discharge.

• If the object is located more posteriorly, is not readily removed on initial attempts, or the patient is completely uncooperative, refer to an otolaryngologist for removal.

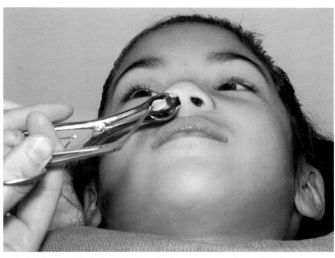

10-2 Removal of foreign body from nose using alligator forceps and nasal speculum.

11. Nasogastric Tube Insertion

PURPOSE: To provide a route for feedings and/or medications or to aspirate stomach contents. This procedure is most often encountered in the operating room, inpatient ward, and emergency room.

EQUIPMENT NEEDED (FIGURE 11-1):

- Gloves
- Towel
- Glass of water with straw
- Emesis basin
- Lubricant
- Topical anesthetic (spray or gel, as desired)
- Goggles
- Catheter tip syringe
- Tape
- Magill forceps
- Wall suction
- Vasoconstrictor nasal spray (e.g., phenylephrine)
- Stethoscope
- 14 to 18F nasogastric (NG) tube (for adults)

TECHNIQUE:

IMPORTANT NOTE: There are two ways of estimating the length of NG tube required for any given patient (about 45 cm). Place the tip of the tubing near the patient's nose, and loop it over the ear and down to about the xiphoid (Figure 11-2). Mark your spot on the tube. The second method is to measure the distance from the ear to the umbilicus. If you are uncertain as to the placement of the tube, check to see if the patient can speak (if not, remove the tube—you are in the trachea).

1. Obtain consent for the procedure from the patient or the next of kin. In a true emergency, a physician may use his or her clinical judgment and place the tube without consent.

2. Have the patient in the sitting position. Place a towel over the patient's chest and place an emesis basin in his or her lap.

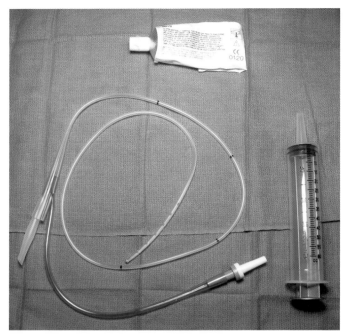

11-1 Equipment for nasogastric tube insertion (from left to right): nasogastric tube, lubricant, catheter tip syringe.

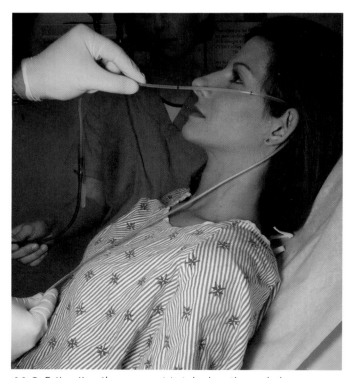

11-2 Estimating the nasogastric tube length needed.

3. Inspect the nares while the patient is inhaling through the nose, and select the most patent one.

4. Place your topical anesthetic of choice (spray or gel) into both nares and the pharynx. Wait enough time for the local anesthetic to work. Size the nostril and choose the largest NG tube that fits within it. If needed, use a topical vasoconstrictor to decrease congestion.

5. Create a curve in the tube (if there is no natural curve) by coiling the first few inches (Figures 11-3a and 11-3b).

6. Prepare the patient for insertion by giving him or her the glass of water to hold.

7. Apply lubricant to the tip of the tube.

8. Hold the patient's head steady and insert the tube by directing it to the floor of the nose (Figure 11-4).

9. Continue advancing the tube until there is resistance (this resistance is most commonly the nasopharynx). Now ask the patient to flex his or her head while swallowing some water through the straw. As soon as the patient swallows, quickly advance the tube into the esophagus. Once there, advance tube smoothly into the stomach (Figure 11-5).

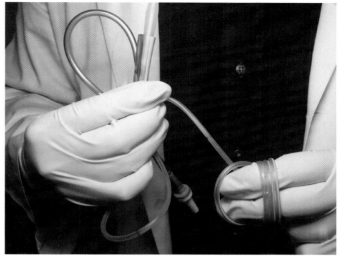

11-3a Wrapping nasogastric tube around fingers.

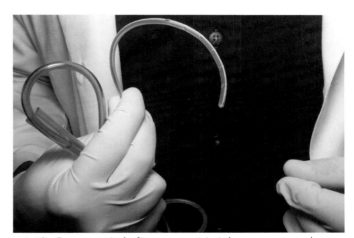

11-3b Curve created after nasogastric tube was wrapped around fingers.

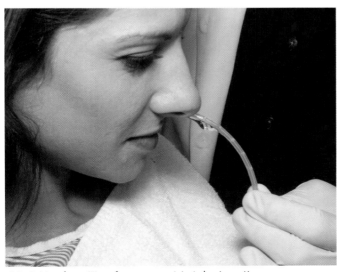

11-4 Head position for nasogastric tube insertion.

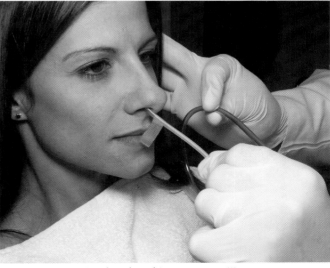

11-5 Nasogastric tube placed in proper position.

10. Watch for immediate return of gastric contents (have emesis basin handy). If you are uncertain, confirm by pushing air with a 60-cc catheter-tip syringe while listening with a stethoscope over the left upper quadrant (LUQ). A "whoosh" sound is heard immediately with proper positioning (Figure 11-6). If the "whoosh" is delayed, the tube may not be in the stomach yet.

11. Secure the tube with tape once you are confident of placement (Figure 11-7).

COMPLICATIONS:

- Epistaxis (if forced)
- Aspiration pneumonia
- Tracheal placement
- Esophageal perforation

POST-PROCEDURE CARE:

1. Monitor electrolytes daily, especially potassium, in cases of prolonged nasogastric suction.

2. Monitor for erosion of nasal, esophageal, or gastric mucosa during long-term use (more than 4 weeks).

PEARLS/TIPS:

- Contraindications include:
    - Suspected cribiform plate injury (facial fractures)
    - Unresponsive patients without a protected airway
    - Esophageal stricture
    - Possible esophageal injury
- In emergencies, most patients tolerate lubrication without local anesthetic (have the emesis basin handy).
- Having the patient flex his or her head helps passing the tube.
- Remember to keep an eye on pressure necrosis of the nose if the tube is to remain for any length of time.

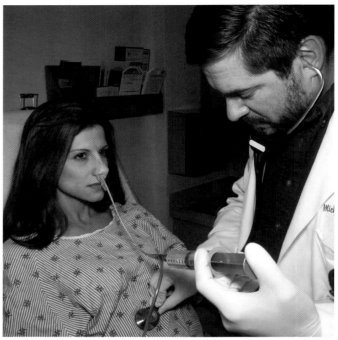

11-6 Listening to determine proper placement of nasogastric tube.

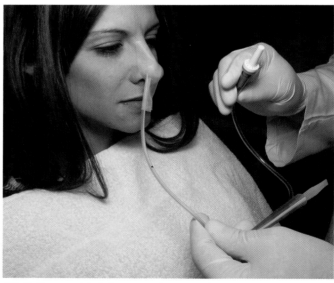

11-7 Nasogastric tube properly secured.

12. Orogastric Tube Insertion

PURPOSE: To provide a route for feedings and/or medications or to aspirate stomach contents. This procedure is most often encountered in the operating room and emergency room. Because an orogastric (OG) tube is far more uncomfortable than an NG tube, usually an OG tube is used only in unresponsive, intubated patients or patients needing gastric lavage in the emergency room.

EQUIPMENT NEEDED:

- Orogastric tube from 50F (for lavage) to 16F (for stomach decompression in the operating room)
- Lubrication (e.g., 2% lidocaine viscous gel)
- Anesthetic spray (topical benzocaine)
- Tongue depressors or curved plastic airway
- Tape
- Eye protection
- Gloves
- Mask
- Gown
- 60-cc syringe

TECHNIQUE # 1—CONSCIOUS PATIENTS:

1. May obtain consent as in step 1 under Technique on page 42.
2. Estimate the amount of OG tube required to reach the stomach (Figure 12-1).
3. Apply topical benzocaine spray to the posterior pharynx.
4. Have the patient flex his or her head forward.
5. Insert tongue depressor or two gloved fingers over the base of the patient's tongue.
6. Guide the OG tube (lubricated) over the dorsal aspect of your fingers or depressor as the patient tries to swallow (Figure 12-2). This may cause some gagging; if so, wait and advance tube immediately after gagging.

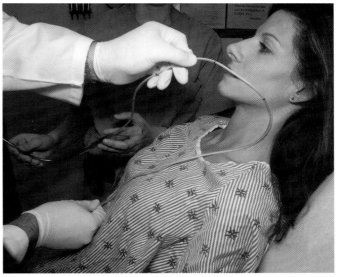

12-1 Estimating the orogastric tube length needed.

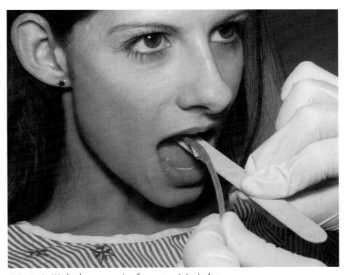

12-2 Initial placement of orogastric tube.

7. Advance tube to previously measured distance (Figure 12-3).

8. Confirm placement by auscultation of the stomach while pushing air with the syringe (Figure 12-4).

9. Secure the tube with tape (Figure 12-5).

TECHNIQUE # 2—OBTUNDED/UNCONSCIOUS PATIENTS:

1. Perform the procedure as above, but use depressors or a curved plastic airway to pull tongue away from posterior pharynx (patient may bite).

COMPLICATIONS:

- Pulmonary aspiration
- Hypoxemia
- Dysrhythmias
- Mucosal injury
- Gastrointestinal tract perforation

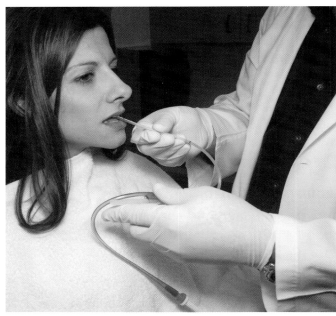

12-3 Orogastric tube inserted.

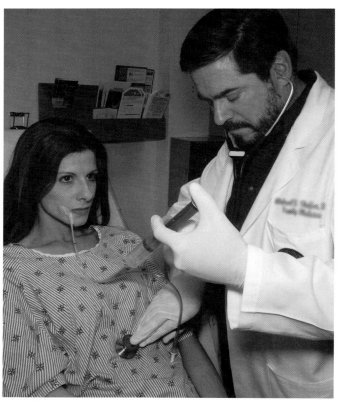

12-4 Listening to determine proper placement of orogastric tube.

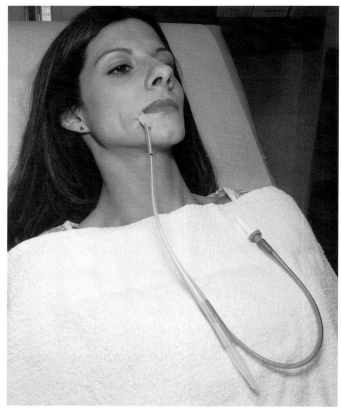

12-5 Orogastric tube properly secured.

POST-PROCEDURE CARE:

1. Reconfirm placement if there is any question of tube location.

PEARLS/TIPS:

- Never forget that an unconscious patient must have an airway secured before attempting placement of gastric tube.

- Waiting to advance tube until after gagging will lessen chance of tracheal placement.

- Remember to keep an eye on pressure necrosis if tube is to remain for any length of time.

13. Endotracheal Intubation

PURPOSE: To secure a patent airway (with obtunded or combative patients) or allow controlled ventilation in patients who are unable to maintain their oxygen saturation (in respiratory failure).

EQUIPMENT NEEDED (FIGURE 13-1):

- Laryngoscope with multiple blades (straight Miller and curved MacIntosh)

- Endotracheal tubes (ETTs) (Sizes 6.5, 7, 7.5, or 8 for adults)

- Malleable stylet (placed in the ETT for improved maneuverability)

- Lubricant for tube

- 10-cc syringe

- Oral airway or bite block

- Tape

- Manual bag and mask

- Ventilator

- Pulse oximeter

- ECG monitor

- Blood pressure monitor

- Yankauer suction

- Crash cart

- Clock

- Stethoscope

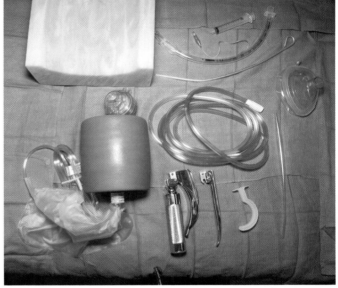

13-1 Equipment for endotracheal intubation: (top) head rest, endotracheal tube, (center, left to right) manual bag and mask, Yankauer suction, face mask, (bottom, left to right) laryngoscope with MacIntosh blade (curved) attached, Miller blade (straight), and oral airway.

- Medications: induction agent (propofol); paralytic (succinylcholine or mivacurium); benzodiazepine (midazolam); narcotic (fentanyl)

- Gloves

- Mask

TECHNIQUE:

> IMPORTANT NOTE: Adept and skillful intubation requires experienced personnel. Always have a backup, preferably an anesthesiologist. Endotracheal intubation is a fairly complex procedure, and whole chapters of textbooks are written to describe proper technique. The basics will be included here.

1. Position the patient supine with head extended and jaw thrust upward off the bed (Figure 13-2).

2. Stand behind the patient's head. The bed's headboard may need to be removed.

3. Apply all monitors (pulse oximeter, ECG leads, and blood pressure cuff).

4. Pre-oxygenate the patient with 100% oxygen for at least 1 minute or four maximal breaths.

5. Make sure all equipment is ready and working. Check the light on the laryngoscope and the cuff on the endotracheal tube by inflating it with 5 cc of sterile water using a syringe. Place the stylet in the ETT and lubricate the ETT tube. Ensure that all personnel are ready.

6. Medicate the patient. Ask the medical or surgical resident what to use and the amount. Anesthetic drugs are dosed on a mg/kg basis. Once patient is paralyzed YOU become his or her lungs.

7. Time yourself or have someone watch the clock. The intubation attempt should not take longer than 20 to 30 seconds (if unsuccessful at this time, stop and ventilate with the mask before second attempt. Have back-up personnel available).

8. Open the patient's mouth by using right index finger on the upper teeth and thumb on lower teeth (Figure 13-3).

9. With left hand holding laryngoscope, place blade of scope on patient's tongue. Have the suction ready. Insert the curved blade into the mouth and pass it into the vallecula (be mindful of the teeth).

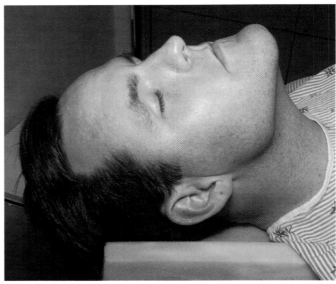

13-2 Proper head position for endotracheal intubation.

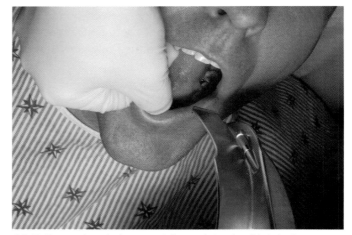

13-3 Proper hand placement for endotracheal intubation.

10. Lift the laryngoscope in a 45° angle in an upward-and-away motion using your shoulder, not your wrist (avoid fulcrum movement).

11. Look for vocal cords (Figures 13-4a and 13-4b). Visualization of cords is crucial to prevent esophageal intubation. If no cords are visible, make sure you are using enough force to pull the jaw and soft tissue up and away from the posterior tissue. Also, an assistant may gently apply cricoid cartilage pressure (Sellick's maneuver) to push cords down into view and help prevent possible aspiration. If cords are still not visible, remove the blade from the patient's mouth and administer 100% oxygen to the patient using the manual bag and valve mask. The patient's position may need to be altered by producing more or less extension of the neck.

12. Keep your eyes fixed down the blade and at the cords. Once you see the cords, have an assistant pass the endotracheal tube to your right hand.

13. Place the ETT through the cords (if apart), making sure that the inflatable ETT cuff is beyond the cords (approximately 18 to 21 cm from the patient's teeth).

14. Keep ETT stabilized with right hand and remove the laryngoscope and the stylet from the ETT (using left hand).

15. Inflate the ETT cuff to approximately 5 cm (if the senescent bag is too hard, you have overinflated the cuff).

16. Ventilate with the manual oxygen bag while auscultating over both upper lung fields and the stomach. Make sure lung sounds are symmetrical and that no sound is heard over the stomach. If asymmetric (right louder than left), you have most probably placed the ETT too deep and entered the right main stem bronchus. Simply withdraw the ETT by 1 cm at a time and auscultate for bilateral equal breath sounds.

17. Connect the ETT to ventilator (ensure correct settings: rate 12 to 20; tidal volume 5–10 cc/kg; and forced inspiration of oxygen [FIO$_2$]) or have an assistant bag-ventilate the patient while you place a curved plastic bite block. Many ETTs now have a CO_2 indicator that allows the physician to confirm placement of the tube in the lungs.

18. Secure tube with tape (noting depth at the teeth).

19. Keep checking the patient's oxygen saturation.

20. Confirm the ETT placement with a stat portable chest x-ray.

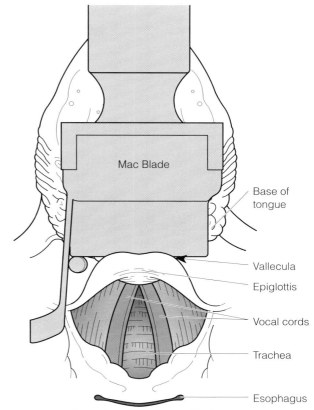

13-4a View of vocal cords with Mac blade.

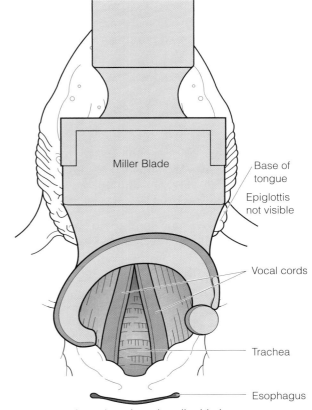

13-4b View of vocal cords with Miller blade.

COMPLICATIONS:

- Throat pain
- Broken teeth
- Arytenoid cartilage dislocation
- Laryngospasm
- Labile blood pressure
- Hypoxia
- Pulmonary aspiration
- Esophageal placement
- Pneumothorax
- Corneal abrasions
- Death

POST-PROCEDURE CARE:

1. Follow placement with daily x-rays of the chest (end of tube should be 2 cm from carina on film).

2. Mismanagement of the airway can be fatal; make certain that the physician who will be responsible for the patient knows about intubation and ventilator settings.

PEARLS/TIPS:

- Use an endotracheal tube size 6.5 to 7.5 for women, and 7.5 to 8.5 for men.

- MacIntosh (curved) blades are easier for inexperienced physicians.

- The position of the patient is very important; make sure the patient is positioned in the "sniffing position" and that the bed is at a comfortable height for you.

- Succinylcholine can cause an increase in serum potassium, so use care with this medication and know the patient's potassium level.

- Avoid damage to the vocal chords by keeping stylet within the ET tube and not extended beyond it.

- If you intubate the esophagus, leave the tube in place, use another ETT and go for the "other" hole, then immediately remove the ETT that was placed in the esophagus.

- Remember the ABCs: a patent *airway* is of the utmost importance in resuscitation of the patient, followed by *breathing* and *circulation*.

IV. Chest and Lungs

14. Central Lines (Venous Access Devices)

The term "central line" typically refers to any venous catheter placed so that the tip of the catheter rests in the large central veins (either the superior vena cava [SVC] or the inferior vena cava [IVC]). The purpose of a central line is to provide IV access when peripheral access is unobtainable or inadequate (e.g., resuscitation efforts, total parenteral nutrition [TPN]), or when the patient requires IV access for a duration of time that makes peripheral access impractical.

Placement

A central line may be placed percutaneously into the subclavian, internal jugular, or femoral veins. A peripherally inserted central catheter is a special type of central line placed into the antecubital fossa, through the basilic or cephalic vein, and with the tip of the catheter resting in the SVC.

Time Frames

A central line may be placed for short-term, intermediate, or long-term access. A short-term central line is any central line intended to stay in place for a period of less than 4 weeks (generally less than 2 weeks). An intermediate central line may stay in place for a period of several weeks to several months. A long-term central line is intended to stay in place for many months to years. Many surgically implanted catheters may be used for either intermediate or long-term access.

Uses

Many short-term central lines are placed solely for the purpose of delivering medications, blood products, or intravenous fluids when a person is hospitalized. Other central lines provide parenteral nutrition to patients either in the hospital or out of the hospital. Central lines placed for parenteral nutrition may be either short-term or intermediate catheters. Central lines may also be placed for delivery of chemotherapy to cancer patients. These lines are usually surgically implanted, semipermanent or permanent central lines, such as an Omegaport. Another use for central lines is for temporary or permanent hemodialysis access. Finally, central lines may be placed for invasive pressure monitoring purposes. A Swan-Ganz catheter is an example of a central line designed for invasive pressure monitoring.

Complications

The complications associated with central line placement vary in seriousness and by location of the central line. Bleeding and infection are the most common complications associated with central lines. Bleeding can occur as a result of the procedure itself (laceration of the vein) or may be related to blood leakage and hematoma formation at the site of the central line. Infections of central lines can range from simple cellulitis or phlebitis to bacterial or fungal sepsis. Thrombosis of the vein in which a central line is placed can occur at any time or in any location. Embolisms may complicate central lines that accidentally rest in the right atrium or ventricle. Pneumothorax or hemothorax is a complication of subclavian and internal jugular central lines. Damage to adjacent nerves, arteries, or solid organs (heart) can occur from any central line placement. An uncommon complication of central lines (particularly Swan-Ganz catheters) is right bundle branch block caused by trauma to the ventricle during central line placement. Hemodialysis catheters and other permanent lines may be predisposed to clotting off the lumen of the catheter and becoming nonfunctional.

Table 14.1 Types of central lines.

Type of Catheter	Comments	Adult or Pediatric	Indication	Temporary or Permanent	# of Lumens	Length	Gauge (ga.) or French (F)	Location of Placement (Subclavian [SC], Internal Jugular [IJ], Femoral)	Type of Procedure (Surgical or Bedside)
Central venous line	Multiple lumens provide for multiple medications or drips at the same IV site	Pediatric	IV access	Temporary	2 lumens	8 cm	22 ga., 4F	SC/Femoral	Bedside
Central venous line		Pediatric	IV access	Temporary	3 lumens	13 cm	22/22/20 ga., 5.5F	SC/Femoral	Bedside
Central venous line		Pediatric	IV access	Temporary	3 lumens	30 cm	22/22/20 ga., 5.5 Fr	Femoral	Bedside
Central venous line		Adult	IV access	Temporary	1 lumen	9 cm	24 ga.	Femoral	Bedside
Central venous line		Pediatric	IV access	Temporary	1 lumen	12 cm	20 ga.	IJ	Bedside
Central venous line		Adult	IV access	Temporary	1 lumen	12 cm	20 ga.	SC/IJ/Femoral	Bedside
Central venous line		Adult	IV access	Temporary	1 lumen	20 cm	16 ga.	SC/IJ/Femoral	Bedside
Central venous line (Figure 14-1)		Adult	IV access	Temporary	3 lumens	20 cm	16/18/18 ga.	SC/IJ/Femoral	Bedside
Central venous line		Adult	IV access	Temporary	3 lumens	16 cm	16/18/18 ga.	SC/IJ/Femoral	Bedside
Central venous line (Figure 14-2)		Adult	IV access	Temporary	2 lumens	16 cm	16/16 ga.	SC/IJ/Femoral	Bedside
Central venous line		Adult	IV access	Temporary	1 lumen	13 cm	20 ga.	SC/IJ/Femoral	Bedside
Percutaneous sheath introducer	May pass a triple lumen catheter or PA catheter through the sheath	Adult	IV access	Temporary	1 lumen w/sideport	N/A	8.5 or 9F	SC/Femoral	Bedside
Percutaneous sheath introducer	Useful for high volume fluid resuscitation or rapid transfusion	Adult	IV access	Temporary	1 lumen w/sideport	10 cm	8.5F	SC/Femoral	Bedside
Hohn percutaneous catheter w/antimicrobial cuff	Antimicrobial cuff allows for more prolonged indwelling than other central lines	Adult	IV access	Temporary	1 lumen	34 cm	5F	SC/IJ	Bedside
Pulmonary artery (PA) catheter (Swan-Ganz)		Adult	Invasive pressure monitoring	Temporary	1 lumen	110 cm	7F	SC/Femoral	Bedside or fluoroscopic
PA catheter (Swan-Ganz) w/CCO and SVO$_2$	CCO = continuous cardiac output, SVO$_2$ = oxygen consumption	Adult	Invasive pressure monitoring	Temporary	1 lumen	110 cm	7.5 or 8F	SC/Femoral	Bedside or fluoroscopic
Introducer for PA catheter (Swan-Ganz) w/multiple IV sites	Allows for both PA catheter and multiple meds or drips	Adult	Invasive pressure monitoring and IV access	Temporary	3 lumens and a port	11 cm	9F	SC	Bedside

Type of Catheter	Comments	Adult or Pediatric	Indication	Temporary or Permanent	# of Lumens	Length	Gauge (ga.) or French (F)	Location of Placement (Subclavian [SC], Internal Jugular [IJ], Femoral)	Type of Procedure (Surgical or Bedside)
Introducer for PA catheter (Swan-Ganz) w/multiple IV sites (Figure 14-3)	Allows for both PA catheter and multiple meds or drips	Adult	Invasive pressure monitoring and IV access	Temporary	2 lumens and a port	10.5 cm	8.5F	SC	Bedside
Introducer for arterial line		Adult	Invasive pressure monitoring	Temporary	1 lumen	12 cm	5 or 6F	Femoral	Bedside
Peripherally inserted central catheter (PICC line) (Figure 14-4)	Allows for more prolonged indwelling than other central lines	Adult/Pediatric	IV access	Temporary	1 or 2 lumens	N/A	18/20/22 ga.	Antecubital fossa	Bedside
Quinton catheter (Figure 14-5)	Acute hemodialysis catheter	Adult/Pediatric	IV access	Temporary	2 lumens	N/A	16 ga.	SC/IJ/Femoral	Bedside
Schon catheter	Hemodialysis catheter	Adult	IV access	Semi-permanent	2 lumens	14 or 16 cm	18/20/22/24F	SC/IJ/Femoral	Surgical
Tesio catheter	Hemodialysis catheter	Adult	IV access	Semi-permanent	2 lumens	N/A	N/A	SC/IJ/Femoral	Surgical
Cook catheter		Adult/Pediatric	IV access	Temporary	1 lumen	8 or 12 cm	3 or 4F	Femoral	Bedside
Hickman catheter	Tunneled catheter	Adult	IV access	Semi-permanent	1, 2, or 3 lumens	N/A	12F	SC/IJ	Surgical
Groshong catheter (Figure 14-6)	Tunneled catheter	Adult	IV access	Semi-permanent	1 or 2 lumens	N/A	7 or 9.5F	SC/IJ	Surgical
Broviac catheter (Figure 14-7)	Tunneled catheter	Adult/Pediatric	IV access	Semi-permanent	1 or 2 lumens	Pedi-2.7 or 4.2 mm, Adult-6.6 mm	N/A	SC/IJ	Surgical
Omegaport, Permacath, others (Figure 14-8)	Subcutaneously placed access with diaphragm set-up, not actual lumens	Adult/Pediatric	IV access, chemotherapy	Permanent	Single diaphragm	Various	Various	SC/IJ	Surgical

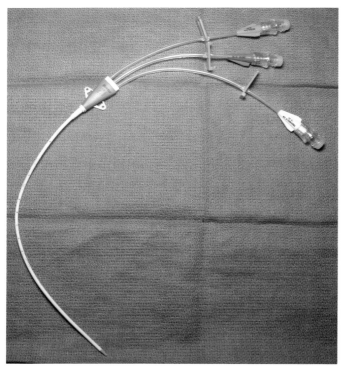

14-1 Triple-lumen catheter.

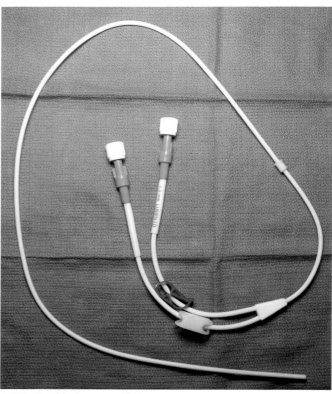

14-2 Double-lumen catheter.

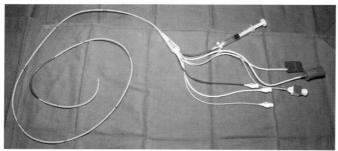

14-3 Swan-Ganz catheter.

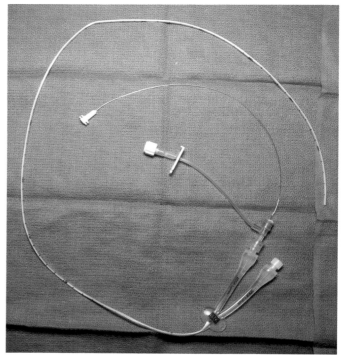

14-4 PICC line.

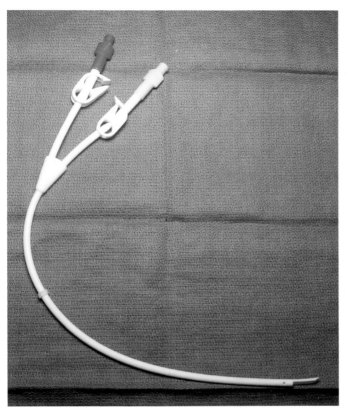

14-5 Quinton catheter.

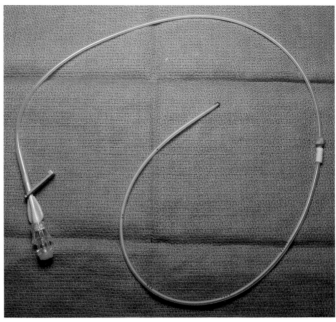

14-6 Groshong catheter.

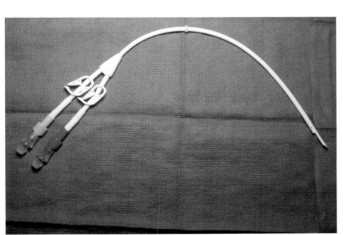

14-7 Broviac catheter.

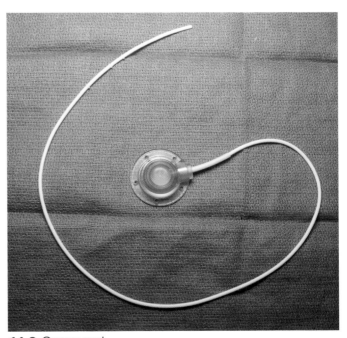

14-8 Omega port.

14a. Subclavian Central Line Placement

PURPOSE: To infuse large volumes of parenteral fluid, monitor central venous pressure, place invasive monitors (Swan-Ganz), create emergency venous access, or administer certain peripheral vascular irritating medications.

EQUIPMENT NEEDED (FIGURE 14-9):

- Sterile gloves
- Sterile gowns
- Sterile towels
- Masks
- Paper hat
- Three 10-cc syringes with saline flush
- Clear semipermeable adhesive film (e.g., Opsite)
- Central venous catheter set that contains a small-gauge needle with syringe for anesthesia; lidocaine 1%; 18-gauge needle with syringe; guide wire; dilator; radiopaque catheter; one IV cap for each access point; 3-0 nylon or silk suture on a straight cutting needle; No. 11 scalpel blade; sterile prep solution; topical antimicrobial ointment; and 4 inch x 4 inch sterile gauze pads.
- Assistant (may be necessary)

TECHNIQUE:

IMPORTANT NOTE: There are two main ways to cannulate the subclavian vein, infraclavicularly and supraclavicularly. The infraclavicular approach using the Seldinger (over guide wire) technique will be discussed here since it is the most commonly used method.

1. Obtain informed consent from the patient or next of kin.

2. Familiarize yourself with the anatomy of the subclavian vein.

3. Place patient in the Trendelenburg's position (head down about 30 degrees), if patient's condition will allow. This may help small or nearly collapsed veins to expand, making cannulation easier and reducing potential complications. Proper positioning of the patient is of the utmost importance.

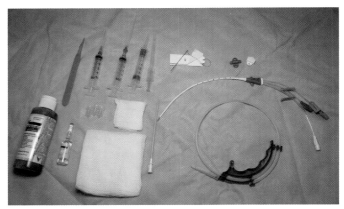

14-9 Equipment for central line placement.

4. Raise the bed height to a comfortable level for you. The patient's arms should be at his or her side and possibly restrained. You may need to have an assistant pull (with constant force) the ipsilateral arm toward the patient's feet. With the patient properly positioned, you are ready to proceed.

5. Observe sterile technique and thoroughly clean the region around the clavicle.

6. Drape the infraclavicular area in a sterile fashion.

7. Orient yourself to the anatomy by feeling the clavicle and sternal notch.

8. Open the kit and place it on a bedside table.

9. Use lidocaine 1% with the small-gauge needle and syringe to anesthetize the skin just below the clavicle.

10. Using the same needle and syringe, continue to use lidocaine 1% to anesthetize the periosteum of the clavicle (remember to aspirate before each injection). You are now done anesthetizing.

11. Attach the 18-gauge needle to the 10-cc syringe included in the kit.

12. Align the bevel of the needle with the markings of the syringe for good technique.

13. Using your nondominant hand re-orient yourself to the landmarks on the patient by placing your thumb over the middle third of the clavicle, and your index finger in the suprasternal notch.

14. Use your dominant hand to insert the 18-gauge needle caudad to the clavicle just medial to the nondominant thumb (Figure 14-10).

15. Advance the needle (aspirating) at a 15° angle relative to the patient's chest wall until the needle touches the patient's clavicle.

16. "Walk" the needle down the clavicle.

17. Decrease the angle of the needle once it is under the clavicle, until it is as parallel to the patient's chest wall as possible.

18. Advance the needle carefully under the clavicle while directing it cephalad toward the suprasternal notch.

19. Maintain constant aspiration while slowly advancing. A sudden flash of dark venous blood will mark your entry into the subclavian vein (about 4 cm) (Figure 14-11). If no flash of blood is seen, withdraw the needle slowly with constant aspiration (you may have gone completely through the vessel). **Note:** If the blood is bright red and pulsatile, you are in the subclavian artery. If in a nonemergency situation, withdraw the needle and apply pressure for 10 minutes.

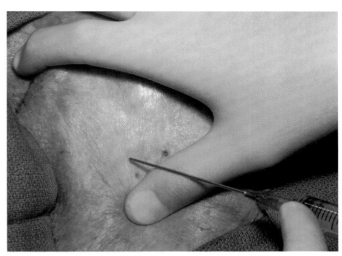

14-10 Insertion point for 18-gauge needle.

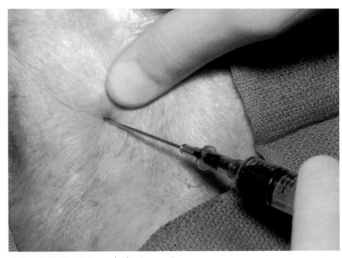

14-11 Entry into subclavian vein.

20. Remove the needle if unsuccessful. Flush the needle to remove any clots or tissue. Repeat the process from steps 19 to 20, but this time redirect the needle slightly cephalad and posterior.

21. Rotate the bevel caudally (this will help the wire pass toward the superior vena cava [SVC] and away from the jugular) once you have successfully entered the subclavian vein (indicated by dark, nonpulsatile blood).

22. Recheck with aspiration that there is still free flow in the needle.

23. Stabilize the needle with your nondominant hand and remove the syringe.

24. Place your thumb over the hub to prevent air emboli.

25. Insert the guide wire smoothly until about 10 cm of it is within the vessel (Figure 14-12).

26. Watch for dysrhythmias (do not irritate those ventricles!).

27. Remove the 18-gauge needle over the wire while keeping the wire firmly in place (an alternative is to keep the needle in place until you have made the incision in the next step, and then remove it [Figure 14-13]).

28. Make a skin incision about the size of the catheter next to the wire (do not cut the wire). *Never* let the wire go free. *Always* have one hand controlling the wire.

29. Thread the dilator (if included) over the wire.

30. Make sure the wire sticks out of the proximal opening of the dilator before releasing the wire near the skin (Figure 14-14).

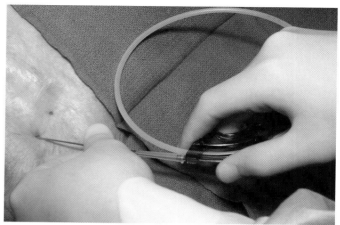

14-12 Insertion of guide wire.

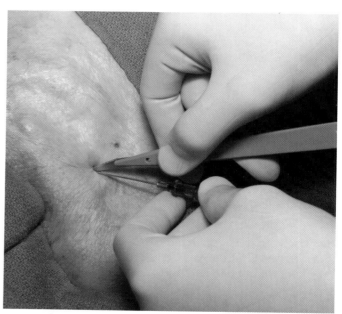

14-13 Skin incision made before dilator placement.

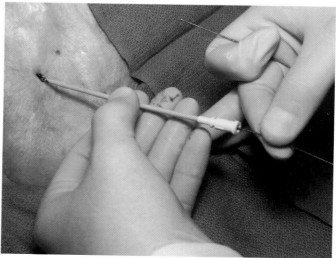

14-14 Threading dilator over guide wire.

31. Hold the wire and advance the dilator over the wire into the subclavian vein (Figure 14-15).

32. Remove the dilator over the wire (keeping the wire in place).

33. Place the catheter (there are multiple types, but the most commonly used is the triple-lumen catheter) over the wire and advance it up to 1 cm from the skin. If resistance occurs, retract the catheter and re-insert.

34. Make sure the wire sticks out of the distal port of the catheter before releasing the wire at the skin (Figure 14-16).

35. Hold the wire firmly at the distal port and advance the catheter while gently twisting. Most catheters are designed to be placed all the way to the hub. However, sometimes it is wise to estimate the length of catheter needed to obtain proper placement in the SVC while the catheter is out of the patient.

36. Remove the wire while holding the catheter firmly in place.

37. Aspirate and flush all the catheter ports once the catheter is in place, and then suture the hub in place with the included 3-0 silk or nylon sutures (Figure 14-17).

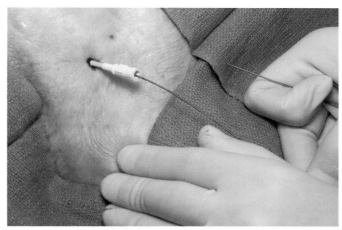
14-15 Complete advancement of dilator.

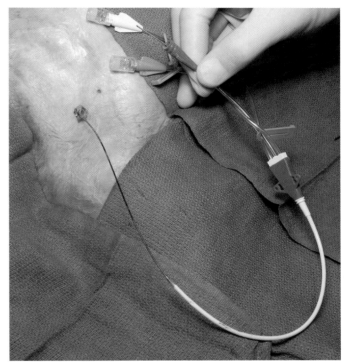
14-16 Threading catheter over guide wire.

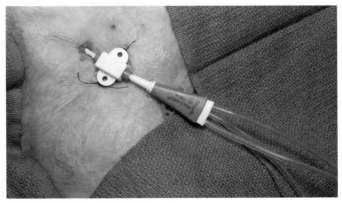
14-17 Catheter sutured into place.

38. Use an antimicrobial: Some suggest using topical antimicrobial ointment on the catheter at the skin and then covering with a clear Opsite. Others use an antimicrobial disk under the Opsite. Doing this may allow you to leave a line in place longer than would normally be tolerated.

39. Obtain a chest x-ray to rule out pneumothorax and ensure proper line placement (line is clear to use if tip is in SVC, but not if going up into the jugular).

COMPLICATIONS:

- Pain
- Bleeding
- Infection
- Hydrothorax
- Pneumothorax
- Hemothorax
- Air embolus
- Nerve injury
- Cardiac dysrhythmias

POST-PROCEDURE CARE:

1. Look at the chest x-ray for the position of the catheter tip and presence of a pneumothorax.

PEARLS/TIPS:

- Contraindications include:
  - Patient refusal
  - Chest deformities
  - Anticoagulation
  - SVC injury
  - Contralateral pneumothorax or hemothorax
- Left versus right? Some advocate using the right subclavian vein because the dome of the pleura of the right lung is usually lower than the left. If you have not gotten blood return on your third attempt, swallow your pride and watch someone else try. Remember, this is a blind stick; no one hits them all the time.

14b. Jugular Central Line Placement

PURPOSE: To infuse large volume parenteral fluid, monitor central venous pressure, place invasive monitors (Swan-Ganz), create emergency venous access, or administer certain peripheral vascular irritating medications.

EQUIPMENT NEEDED:

- Sterile gloves
- Sterile gowns
- Sterile towels
- Mask
- Paper hat
- Three 10-cc syringes with saline flush
- Clear semipermeable adhesive film (e.g., Opsite)
- Central venous catheter set that contains a small-gauge needle with syringe for anesthesia; lidocaine 1%; 18-gauge needle with syringe; guide wire; dilator; radiopaque catheter; one IV cap for each access point; 3-0 nylon or silk suture on a straight cutting needle; No. 11 scalpel blade; sterile prep solution; topical antimicrobial ointment; and 4 inch $\times$ 4 inch sterile gauze pads.

TECHNIQUE:

IMPORTANT NOTE: This procedure is very similar to the insertion of a subclavian catheter. There are multiple ways to perform this procedure, but the central approach, using the Seldinger (over the wire) technique, will be shown here. Know your anatomy! If you know nothing else, know that the carotid artery is medial to the jugular vein. There are different methods in obtaining access to the internal jugular. Some use the 18-gauge needle; others use a catheter-over-needle device; and still others use a small "finder" needle (22-gauge) to locate the jugular, then use the larger needle along the same path as the finder.

1. Obtain informed consent from the patient or next of kin.

2. Orient yourself to the anatomy by feeling for the carotid artery. The jugular vein will be lateral to the carotid artery.

3. Observe sterile technique. Sterile preparation of the patient is important. Also, have the central line kit open and ready to use.

4. Palpate the triangle formed by the clavicle and the two heads of the sternocleidomastoid muscle with your left index finger (Figure 14-18).

5. Palpate the right carotid artery, which is posteromedial to the jugular vein (Figure 14-19).

6. Use 1% lidocaine to anesthetize the skin just caudad to the apex of the triangle formed by the two heads of the sternocleidomastoid muscle if needed.

7. Remember to aspirate before each injection of local as you anesthetize the deeper tissue toward the ipsilateral nipple (which is parallel to the course of the carotid artery) with an angle of about 40 degrees to the horizontal plane of the patient. You are now finished anesthetizing.

8. Attach the 18-gauge needle to the 10-cc syringe included in the kit.

9. Place your nondominant hand over the carotid to prevent you from attempting to move the needle too medially.

10. Aspirate with the syringe while slowly advancing the needle.

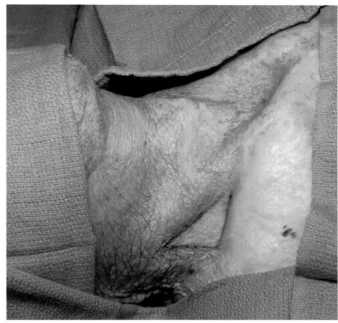

14-18 Triangle formed by the clavicle and the two heads of the sternocleidomastoid muscle.

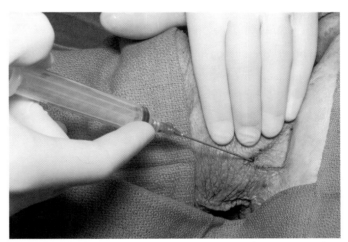

14-19 Palpation of carotid artery, as needle is being inserted, helps prevent accidentally puncturing the carotid artery.

11. Watch for dark venous blood return (at about 2 to 3 cm), as with the subclavian technique (Figure 14-20). If no blood returns, slowly pull needle back (no need to completely remove the needle) and reposition, angling slightly lateral to initial attempt. **Note:** If bright red, pulsating blood returns, and the situation is not emergent, remove needle and apply pressure for 20 minutes.

12. Ensure the needle is completely within jugular vein when dark blood returns, by rotating the bevel while aspirating slightly.

13. Stabilize the needle with your nondominant hand and remove the syringe.

14. Place your thumb over the hub to prevent air emboli.

15. Insert the guide wire smoothly until about 10 cm of it is within the vessel (Figure 14-21).

16. Remove the 18-gauge needle over the wire while keeping the wire firmly in place (an alternative is to keep the needle in place until you have made the incision in the next step, and then remove it).

17. Make a skin incision about the size of the catheter next to the wire (do not cut the wire). *Never* let the wire go free. *Always* have one hand controlling the wire.

18. Thread the dilator (if included) over the wire.

19. Make sure the wire sticks out of the proximal opening of the dilator before releasing the wire near the skin.

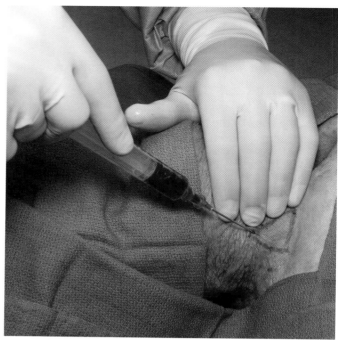

14-20 Entry into jugular vein.

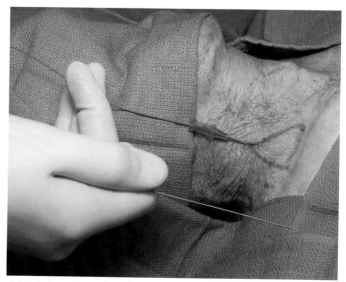

14-21 Insertion of guide wire into jugular vein.

20. Hold the wire and advance the dilator over the wire into the jugular vein (Figure 14-22).

21. Remove the dilator over the wire (keeping the wire in place).

22. Place the catheter (there are multiple types, but the most commonly used is the triple-lumen catheter) over the wire and advance it up to 1 cm from the skin. If resistance is felt, retract the catheter and re-insert.

23. Make sure the wire sticks out of the distal port of the catheter before releasing the wire at the skin (Figure 14-23).

24. Hold the wire firmly at the distal port and advance the catheter while gently twisting. Most catheters are designed to be placed all the way to the hub. However, sometimes it is wise to estimate the length of catheter needed to obtain proper placement in the superior vena cava (SVC) while the catheter is out of the patient.

25. Remove the wire while holding the catheter firmly in place.

26. Aspirate and flush all ports of the catheter once in place, and then suture the hub in place with the included 3-0 silk or nylon sutures (Figure 14-24).

27. Use an antimicrobial: Some suggest using topical antimicrobial ointment on the catheter at the skin and then covering with a clear Opsite. Others use an antimicrobial disk under the Opsite. Doing this may allow you to leave a line in place longer than would normally be tolerated.

28. Obtain a chest x-ray to check the catheter tip position.

COMPLICATIONS:
- Pain, bleeding
- Infection
- Air embolus
- Nerve injury
- Cardiac dysrhythmias

POST-PROCEDURE CARE:

1. Check the chest x-ray for catheter tip position.

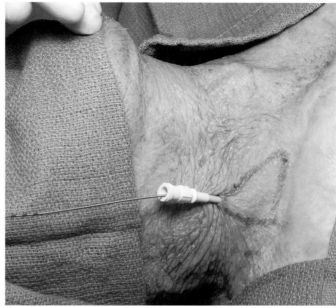

14-22 Complete advancement of dilator.

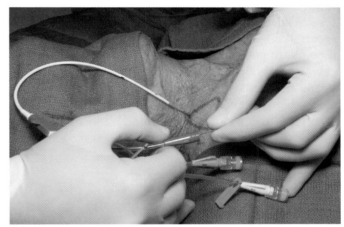

14-23 Threading catheter over guide wire.

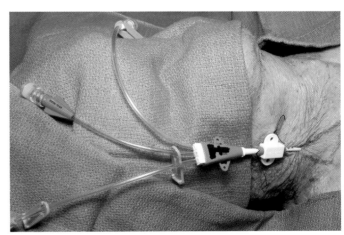

14-24 Catheter sutured into place.

PEARLS/TIPS:

- Contraindications include:
  - Patient refusal
  - Anticoagulation
  - SVC injury

- If you apply constant pressure to the carotid, you may decrease the diameter of the internal jugular.

- Using a finder needle can save you if you accidentally puncture the carotid.

14c. Femoral Central Line Placement

PURPOSE: To gain access to the circulatory system when the patient has no other access sites, or when it is difficult to obtain access elsewhere in an emergency. There are several advantages to using the femoral vein for central access: It is fast and easy with a higher success rate, there is no risk of pneumothorax, and it does not interfere with airway placement and management. However, there are disadvantages to consider also: It takes longer for drugs to reach central circulation during cardiopulmonary resuscitation (CPR), it prevents patient mobilization, and there is a higher risk of infection and higher incidence of deep vein thrombosis.

EQUIPMENT NEEDED:

- Sterile gloves
- Sterile gowns
- Sterile towels
- Masks
- Paper hat
- Three 10-cc syringes with saline flush
- Clear semipermeable adhesive film (e.g., Opsite)
- Central venous catheter set that contains the following: small-gauge needle with syringe for anesthesia; lidocaine 1%; 18-gauge needle with syringe; guide wire; dilator; radiopaque catheter; one IV cap for each access point; 3-0 nylon or silk suture on a straight cutting needle; No. 11 blade; sterile prep solution; topical antimicrobial ointment; and 4 inch × 4 inch sterile gauze pads.

TECHNIQUE:

IMPORTANT NOTE: The approach using the Seldinger (over guide wire) technique will be discussed here.

1. Obtain informed consent from the patient or next of kin.

2. Orient yourself to the anatomy by feeling for the femoral artery pulsation. The femoral vein will be medial to the femoral artery (Figure 14-25).

3. Observe sterile technique and thoroughly clean the region around the groin.

4. Drape the area in a sterile fashion.

5. Open the kit and place it on a bedside table.

6. Use the small-gauge needle to anesthetize the skin (remember to aspirate before each injection) (Figure 14-26). You are now done anesthetizing.

7. Palpate the femoral artery with your finger and insert the 18-gauge needle (attached to the 10-cc syringe) approximately 1 cm medial to the artery (Figure 14-27).

8. Insert the needle at a 30° to 45° angle approximately 1 cm below the inguinal ligament.

9. Direct the needle toward the umbilicus.

10. Position the dominant hand so the syringe's piston can be withdrawn slightly, creating a negative pressure in the cylinder.

11. Maintain constant aspiration while slowly advancing. A sudden flash of dark venous blood will mark your entry into the femoral vein (Figure 14-28). **Note:** If the blood is bright red and pulsatile, you are in the femoral artery. If this happens in a nonemergency, withdraw the needle and apply pressure for 10 minutes.

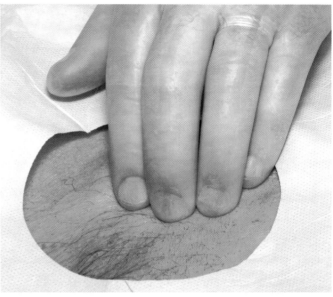

14-25 Palpation of femoral artery.

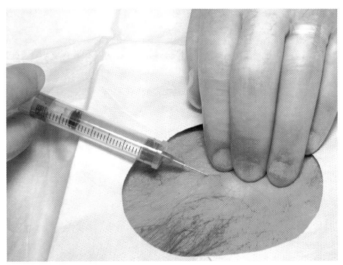

14-26 Superficial anesthetization of the skin.

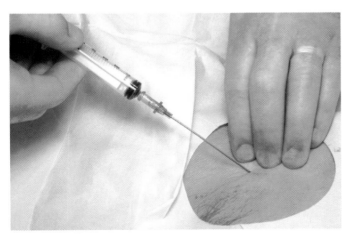

14-27 Needle insertion.

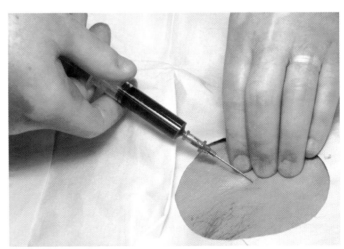

14-28 Entry into the femoral vein.

12. Stabilize the needle with your nondominant hand and remove the syringe.

13. Place your thumb over the hub to prevent air emboli.

14. Insert the guide wire smoothly until about 10 cm is within the vessel (Figure 14-29).

15. Remove the 18-gauge needle over the wire while keeping the wire firmly in place.

16. Make a skin incision about the size of the catheter next to the wire (do not cut the wire) (Figure 14-30). *Never* let the wire go free. *Always* have one hand controlling the wire.

17. Thread the dilator (if included) over the wire.

18. Make sure the wire sticks out of the proximal opening of the dilator before releasing the wire near the skin.

19. Hold the wire and advance the dilator over the wire into the femoral vein (Figure 14-31).

20. Remove the dilator over the wire, keeping the wire in place.

21. Place the catheter (there are multiple types, but the most commonly used is the triple-lumen catheter) over the wire and advance up to 1 cm from the skin.

22. Make sure the wire sticks out of the distal port of the catheter before releasing the wire at the skin.

23. Hold the wire firmly at the distal port and advance the catheter while gently twisting. If any resistance is met, retract the catheter and re-insert. Most catheters are designed to be placed all the way to the hub (Figure 14-32).

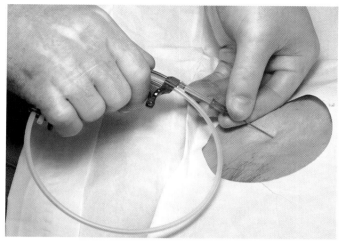

14-29 Insertion of guide wire into femoral vein.

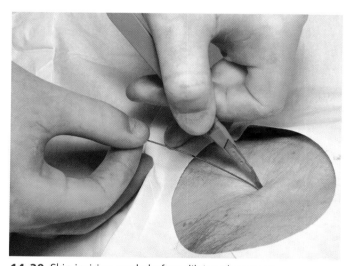

14-30 Skin incision made before dilator placement.

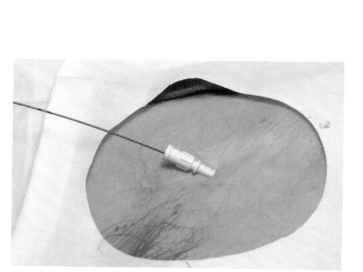

14-31 Complete advancement of dilator.

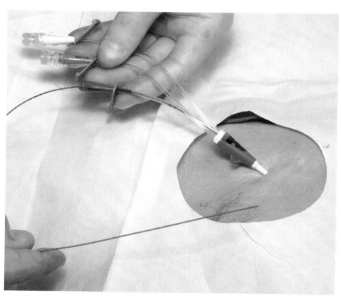

14-32 Threading catheter over guide wire.

24. Remove the wire while holding the catheter firmly in place.

25. Aspirate and flush all ports of the catheter once it is in place, then suture the hub in place with the included 3-0 silk or nylon sutures.

26. Use an antimicrobial: Some suggest using topical antimicrobial ointment on the catheter at the skin and then covering with a clear Opsite. Others use an antimicrobial disk under the Opsite. Doing this may allow you to leave a line in place longer than would normally be tolerated.

COMPLICATIONS:

- Pain
- Bleeding
- Infection

POST-PROCEDURE CARE:

1. Make sure site is appropriately dressed and kept clean to decrease the risk of infection.

2. Remove the catheter as soon as possible because of the potential complications of femoral catheter placement, such as increased risk of infection because of close proximity to genital area.

PEARLS/TIPS:

- Contraindications include:
  - IVC filter
  - Femoral or vena caval thrombosis
  - Absent femoral pulse
  - Penetrating abdominal trauma
  - Cardiac arrest or low flow rates
  - Requirements for patient mobility
- Do not leave the catheter in for longer than 24 hours because of the possibility of thrombosis formation.
- Locate the femoral artery with a Doppler flow detector, then place a mark on the site of the femoral artery. This may be useful if palpation of the artery is difficult.
- Never insert a needle above the inguinal ligament to avoid needle insertion into the abdominal cavity.

15. Swan-Ganz (Pulmonary Artery) Catheter Placement

PURPOSE: Entire chapters have been written on the pulmonary artery (PA) catheter, or Swan-Ganz, listing the many indications, both diagnostic and therapeutic. Briefly, the Swan-Ganz catheter allows invasive monitoring of the pressures within the vasculature for calculations of the patient's hemodynamic status.

EQUIPMENT NEEDED:

- Swan-Ganz catheter (see Figure 14-3)
- Transducer
- Pressure tubing
- Bedside monitor
- Sterile gowns
- Sterile drapes
- Sterile gloves
- Masks
- Paper hat
- Central venous access
- 7F pulmonary artery thermodilution catheter with syringe for balloon
- At least one assistant
- Crash cart readily available

TECHNIQUE:

IMPORTANT NOTE: Before one can place a PA catheter, a central line with a port for this catheter must be in place.

1. Have an assistant calibrate and level the transducer.

2. Observe strict sterile technique.

3. Remove the Swan-Ganz catheter and flush all ports with sterile heparinized saline.

4. Check the small balloon with the included syringe (some suggest testing for air leaks by submerging the balloon in sterile saline and watching for bubbles).

5. Give the proximal end of the catheter to your assistant, while the distal end remains with you on the sterile field.

6. Have your assistant connect the tubing to the ports, and once again test the patency of the ports by having him or her flush the ports.

7. Place the catheter's expanding sheath over the Swan-Ganz catheter for later use.

8. Put the distal end of the Swan-Ganz catheter into the port on the central line in the patient (an 8.5F line in most cases).

9. Pass the catheter tip, with balloon deflated, through the central line to the 10-cm mark on the Swan-Ganz catheter.

10. Observe the waveform on the monitor for the central venous tracing and make sure that the monitor is set to the appropriate scale by your assistant.

11. Have your assistant inflate the balloon. The balloon will act as a sail and help the catheter to advance in the direction of blood flow.

12. Advance the Swan-Ganz to the 30-cm mark in a fluid motion while watching the pressure monitor for the characteristic right ventricular tracing.

13. Watch for ventricular ectopy. If a sustained ventricular arrhythmia occurs, deflate the balloon and withdraw the Swan-Ganz.

14. Identify the ventricular tracing, and then quickly advance to around the 45-cm mark. This should place the distal tip of the Swan-Ganz into the PA. Now is the time for you to slow down the advancement of the catheter.

15. Continue advancing the catheter to approximately 50 cm. There will be a loss of the PA tracing. At this point, stop advancement of the catheter. You have essentially occluded the PA and obtained your pulmonary capillary wedge pressure, which is actually nothing more than the reading of pressure reflected back from the left atrium.

16. Obtain the wedge pressure, then have your assistant deflate the balloon while you watch for the return of the PA tracing.

17. Extend the catheter's expanding sheath from the proximal end to the port on the central line (this allows future adjustment of the Swan-Ganz catheter while maintaining sterile conditions within the expanding sheath).

18. Dress the site and order a chest x-ray.

COMPLICATIONS:

- Ventricular ectopy
- Kinking of catheter
- Vessel puncture
- Embolism
- Balloon rupture
- Endocarditis
- Valve damage
- Catheter fracture

POST-PROCEDURE CARE:

1. Obtain a chest x-ray. Most correct placements of a PA catheter leave the distal tip about 3 to 4 cm from the midline on x-ray.

PEARLS/TIPS:

- Think of the Swan-Ganz pulmonary artery catheter as a sailboat. The sail (balloon) must be raised to move forward. The sail (balloon) must be lowered to be pulled backwards.

- *Never* pull the PA catheter backwards with the balloon inflated, because you could damage valves.

16. Chest Tube Placement

PURPOSE: To remove fluid (hemothorax, chylothorax, empyema) or air (pneumothorax) from the pleural space.

EQUIPMENT NEEDED (FIGURE 16-1):

- Sterile gown
- Sterile gloves
- Mask
- Cap
- Antiseptic solution
- Chest tube
- Petrolatum-impregnated gauze
- Tape
- Wall suction
- Clear tubing
- Thoracostomy tray: lidocaine 1%, 10-cc syringe, 22- and 25-gauge needles, sterile towels, basin, sterile 4 inch × 4 inch gauze pads, straight scissors, curved scissors, clamps, needle holder, 2-0 nonabsorbable sutures on large cutting needles, No. 10 or No. 11 scalpel, forceps
- Sterile drapes
- Suction-drainage system (classic example is the three-bottle system)

TECHNIQUE:

1. Obtain informed consent from the patient or next of kin.

2. Select the correct chest tube size (18 to 20F for pneumothorax, 32 to 40F for fluid or blood).

3. Make sure the suction-drain system is set up and ready to be used.

4. Connect the suction-drain system to a wall suction outlet.

5. Adjust suction until a steady stream of bubbles is produced in the water column.

6. Position the patient supine with the head of the bed slightly elevated (about 45 degrees) and the patient's arm on the affected side placed over his or her head.

7. Follow universal precautions for blood and body fluid exposure.

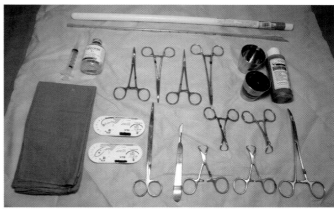

16-1 Equipment for chest tube placement.

8. Make certain that everything remains sterile (wear cap, gloves, and gown).

9. Mark your sight of entry (for the *pleural insertion site*, not the *skin incision site*) with your fingernail or skin marker. The most common site is the mid- to anterior axillary line lateral to about the nipple line—this should avoid the diaphragm.

10. Use sterile technique to arrange your instruments, and prep the patient with the antiseptic solution.

11. Find the rib beneath your *pleural insertion site*.

12. Anesthetize the insertion site with lidocaine using a small-gauge (22- or 25-gauge) needle (Figure 16-2).

13. Anesthetize all the way to the rib, and once the rib is touched continue anesthetizing as you "walk" your needle up over the superior aspect of the rib (Figure 16-3).

14. Anesthetize the parietal pleura and advance slightly while aspirating to check for fluid or air (if none, move one rib superior).

15. Move to your *skin incision site*. Do not get confused here; your *pleural insertion site* is one rib superior to your *skin incision site*, once your pleural insertion site is anesthetized.

16. Make a skin wheal at the *skin incision site* (some feel it good practice to anesthetize from the skin incision wheal up toward your pleural insertion site).

17. Make a transverse 2- to 4-cm incision at the *skin incision site*, through the skin and deeper tissues over the rib (Figure 16-4).

18. Dissect, by blunt Kelly clamp, down to the fascia overlying the intercostal muscle just superior to the rib you chose as your *pleural insertion site* (Figure 16-5).

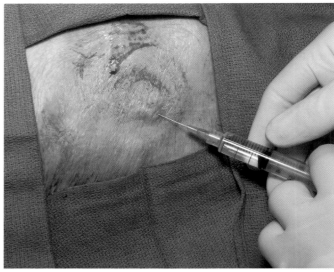
16-2 Anesthetization at the insertion site.

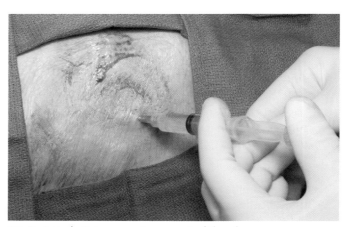
16-3 Anesthetizing superior aspect of the rib.

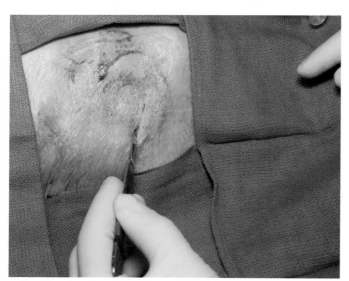
16-4 The skin incision site.

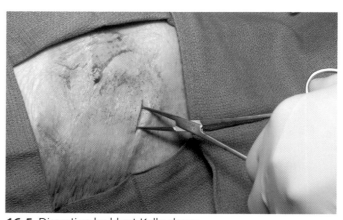
16-5 Dissection by blunt Kelly clamp.

19. Use the closed Kelly clamp to push through the parietal pleura with steady pressure once your *pleural insertion site* has been reached (Figure 16-6). As soon as you feel the clamp push through the parietal pleura, open the clamp widely and withdraw (fluid or air will rush out).

20. Insert a gloved index finger and feel to make sure you have entered the pleural space and that you are clear of any obstacles such as the diaphragm.

21. Grasp the chest tube with a Kelly clamp (make sure the tip of the chest tube protrudes just beyond the end of the clamp).

22. Make sure to clamp the free end of the chest tube to prevent back flow once inserted.

23. Place the chest tube into the pleural space using the finger you left inside the pleural space as a guide (Figure 16-7). The direction you choose to guide the chest tube depends on the patient's pathology. For a pneumothorax, guide the tip of the tube superiorly. For fluid drainage, direct the tip of the tube medially and posteriorly.

24. Once placed, connect the free, clamped end to the suction-drainage system.

25. Check the patency of the system by having the patient cough and watching for a change in the water column level (or bubbles).

26. Secure the chest tube in place, using a large (1-0 or 2-0) nonabsorbable suture. There are multiple ways to secure the chest tube, so ask your resident which they prefer. Here is a common method:

    a. Place the first suture next to the tube and tie off, leaving both ends long (Figure 16-8).

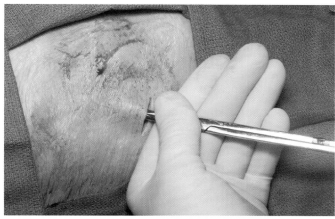

16-6 Using the closed Kelly clamp to push through the parietal pleura.

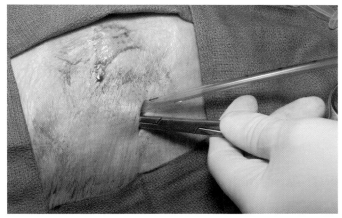

16-7 Placement of the tube into the pleural space.

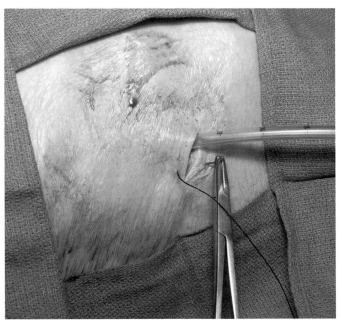

16-8 Placement of the first suture next to the tube.

b. Twist the long ends upward around the chest tube in opposite directions (Figure 16-9).

c. Tie the ends securely.

d. Make sure the chest tube is well anchored, and then close the incision around the anchored chest tube.

e. Use a purse-string stitch around the tube and close the skin tightly around the tube.

f. Dress the site with a petrolatum-impregnated gauze (by wrapping the gauze around the tube at the skin) and 4 inch × 4 inch sterile gauze pads (Figure 16-10).

g. Tape the tube securely to the patient's side.

h. Order an upright and lateral chest x-ray to confirm placement of tube.

COMPLICATIONS:

- Pneumothorax
- Intercostal artery injury
- Infection
- Pain
- Diaphragm injury

POST-PROCEDURE CARE:

1. Make sure to check the x-ray to confirm placement.

2. Chest tubes are usually removed when less than 100 cc of output has been recorded in the last 24 hours.

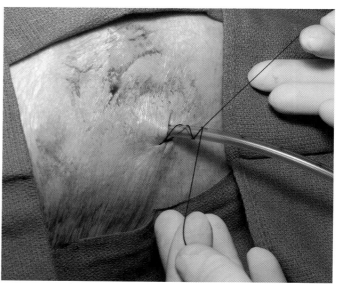

16-9 Twist the long ends upward around the chest tube.

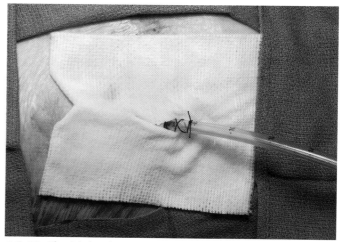

16-10 Chest tube dressing.

PEARLS/TIPS:

- Contraindications include:
  - Patient refusal
  - Anticoagulation
  - Loculated pneumothorax or hydrothorax
  - Previous pleural scarring

- Where to stick? Your *skin incision site* will be about 1 rib below your *pleural insertion site* (which is usually even with the nipple in males).

- When cleaning the patient, a larger area than you feel you need is best.

- Avoid the liver and spleen by properly positioning the patient and knowing as much as possible about the patient's anatomy (prior x-ray could be helpful).

17. Thoracentesis

PURPOSE: To remove fluid from the pleural "space" (a potential space between visceral and parietal pleura). Indications include pleural effusions.

EQUIPMENT NEEDED (FIGURE 17-1):

- Sterile gauze pads
- Tape
- Sterile gloves
- Mask
- Sterile towels
- Povidone iodine solution (Betadine)
- 10-cc 1% lidocaine with epinephrine
- 25-gauge needle
- 22-gauge needle
- 1-inch 15-gauge needle
- 2-inch 15- or 18-gauge needle (15 for fluid, 18 for air)
- 10-cc Luer-Lok syringe
- 50-cc Luer-Lok syringe
- Three-way stopcock
- Clamps
- Sterile plastic tubing
- 1000-cc vacuum bottle
- Oxygen via nasal cannula

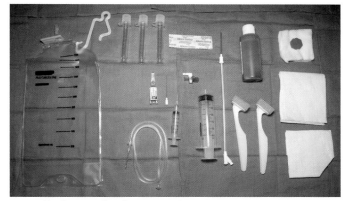

17-1 Equipment for thoracentesis.

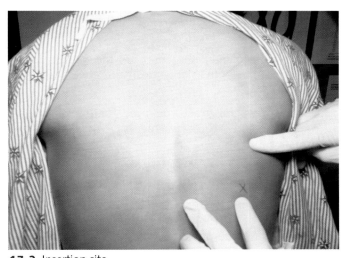

17-2 Insertion site.

TECHNIQUE:

1. Position the patient. Have the patient sit on edge of bed and lean forward onto a bedside table.

2. Mark your insertion site by percussion, x-ray, ultrasound, and/or auscultation.

3. Use the area one or two spaces below the fluid level and 5 to 10 cm lateral to the spine (*not* below the eighth intercostal space) (Figure 17-2).

4. Sterilize the skin with a solution such as Betadine.

5. Use sterile technique, wear a mask, and observe universal precautions.

6. Use lidocaine with epinephrine to raise a skin wheal with a 25-gauge needle.

7. Change to a longer, larger needle (i.e., 1 1/2-inch 22-gauge).

8. Anesthetize the deeper tissue by angling the needle slightly downward through the skin wheal.

9. Aim for the superior border of the rib (always avoid the vein, artery, and nerve that runs along the inferior aspect of each rib).

10. Aspirate and inject local as you advance by "walking" the needle over the superior margin of the rib.

11. Continue to "walk" the needle up into the interspace and confirm the presence of fluid once the parietal pleura has been penetrated (a "pop" may be felt).

12. Place a clamp on the needle at the skin level to mark the depth.

13. Prepare your 50-cc syringe with a three-way stopcock and attach a large-gauge needle (15 for liquid, 18 for air).

14. Make sure to mark the depth on the needle with a clamp (same depth as on your small-gauge anesthesia needle).

15. Follow the same tract you used for the anesthesia needle (Figure 17-3), and advance until the clamp touches the skin.

16. Make sure the stopcock is open to the syringe, and aspirate to confirm placement (fluid should return).

17. Attach one end of the tubing to the stopcock and the other end of the tubing to a needle (to be placed into an evacuated container). Once the needle is in the evacuated container, it is safe to open the stopcock to the needle in the chest.

18. Withdraw the thoracentesis needle (while the patient is exhaling) when the desired amount of fluid has been removed (usually less than 1 liter; 100 mL for diagnostic tests).

19. Clean and dress the site.

20. Order a chest x-ray to rule out pneumothorax.

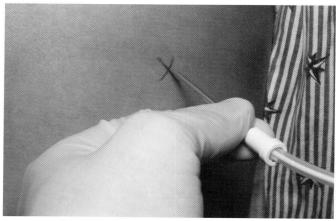

17-3 Needle insertion.

COMPLICATIONS:

- Pneumothorax

- Hemothorax (avoid inferior border of rib)

- Organ damage (be certain of fluid level, and avoid spleen, diaphragm, and liver)

- Re-expansion pulmonary edema (most common if large volumes are removed rapidly)

- Hypoxia (use oxygen for a few hours after procedure)

- Dry tap

- Pain

- Bleeding

- Infection

- Hypovolemia

POST-PROCEDURE CARE:

1. Obtain a stat chest x-ray to check for pneumothorax.

2. Check labs for fluid results (protein and LDH of fluid and plasma are the most common labs) to determine whether the fluid is an exudate or transudate. This is helpful in diagnosing the cause of a pleural effusion.

PEARLS/TIPS:

- Contraindications include:

  - Patient refusal

  - Coagulopathy

  - Insertion site infection

- Warn the patient that some pain can be experienced as the needle passes through the pleura.

- Some patients will not tolerate a therapeutic thoracentesis that removes greater than 1 liter of fluid.

- If you think that you will order more tests later, make sure the lab saves the remainder of the fluid.

18. Rapid Reduction of Tension Pneumothorax (Needle Decompression)

PURPOSE: To relieve the pressure of a tension pneumothorax. Symptoms include dyspnea in a conscious patient, unilateral rise and fall of the chest, absent or decreased breath sounds unilaterally, and hyper-resonance to percussion unilaterally.

EQUIPMENT NEEDED:

- 14 gauge over the IV needle catheter (or through-the-needle catheter)

- 10-cc syringe filled with sterile saline

- Piece of Penrose drain tubing attached to a cut-off 10-cc syringe

- Suture

TECHNIQUE:

1. Find the third rib, mid-clavicular line.

2. Insert the 14-gauge needle (attached to the 10-cc syringe filled with saline) perpendicularly in the mid-clavicular line over the upper edge of the rib (Figure 18-1).

3. Once the rib is felt, "walk" the needle over the superior aspect of the rib and into the lower portion of the second intercostal space.

4. Aspirate the syringe gently as you advance the needle. A "pop" may be felt as the needle enters the pleural space and air is encountered; there will be bubbles in the syringe.

5. Advance the catheter fully into the thorax through the needle.

6. Withdraw the needle and attach the Penrose drain attached to the cut-off 10-cc syringe to serve as a one-way drainage device if needed.

7. Suture the catheter to the chest wall.

COMPLICATIONS:

- Pneumothorax

- Hemothorax (avoid inferior border of rib)

- Organ damage (be certain of fluid level, and avoid spleen, diaphragm, and liver)

- Hypoxia (use oxygen for a few hours after procedure)

- Pain

- Bleeding

- Infection

POST-PROCEDURE CARE:

1. Obtain a stat chest x-ray to check for pneumothorax.

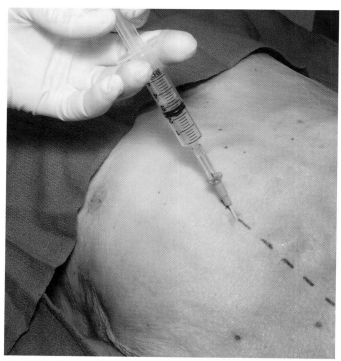

18-1 Site for needle insertion to reduce tension pneumothorax.

PEARLS/TIPS:

- Warn the patient that some pain can be experienced as the needle passes through the pleura.

V. Heart and Peripheral Vasculature

19. Electrocardiogram

PURPOSE: To help diagnose the presence or absence of heart disease, including coronary, valvular, or rhythm disturbances.

EQUIPMENT NEEDED:

- ECG machine
- Conduction pads

TECHNIQUE:

1. Arrange the patient in the supine position.

2. Place conduction pads on the proper positions on the patient (Figure 19-1).

3. Clip limb electrodes onto the conduction pads on the wrists and ankles (more proximal placement is fine).

4. Place anterior chest leads. Clip the leads onto the conduction pads (Figure 19-1):

    a. V1: fourth intercostal space at the right sternal border

    b. V2: fourth intercostal space at the left sternal border

    c. V3: between V2 and V4

    d. V4: fifth intercostal space at midclavicular line (just below the nipple)

    e. V5: anterior axillary line lateral to V4

    f. V6: midaxillary line lateral to V5

5. Set the machine in the run mode.

COMPLICATIONS:

- Local skin irritation

POST-PROCEDURE CARE:

1. Base follow-up treatment on the results of the ECG.

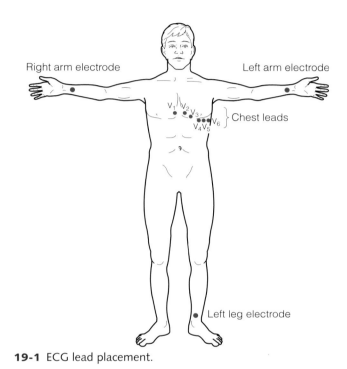

19-1 ECG lead placement.

- May have to shave areas if hair interferes with tracing.
- Most ECG machines have useful directions clearly displayed.

20. Pericardiocentesis

PURPOSE: Percutaneous removal of pericardial fluid from a patient with a pericardial effusion. Usually done with ultrasound guidance, although a blind approach can be done in emergencies or when ultrasound is not available. Signs of significant pericardial effusion include pulsus paradoxus, or enlarged heart with water bottle configuration determined from a chest x-ray.

EQUIPMENT NEEDED:

- 18- to 20-gauge cardiac needle or long central venous catheter with needle
- Povidone iodine (Betadine) or other antiseptic
- Electrocardiogram (ECG) monitor
- No. 11 scalpel blade
- Local anesthetic

TECHNIQUE:

1. Attach electrocardiogram to patient.
2. Arrange the patient so his or her head is elevated at a 30° to 45° angle.
3. Anesthetize site and make a small incision with No. 11 blade.
4. Insert needle subxiphoid and direct toward the left shoulder, aspirating while advancing (Figure 20-1).
5. Continue until fluid is obtained (Figure 20-2).

COMPLICATIONS:

- Laceration of coronary vessels
- Cardiac laceration
- Bleeding
- Dysrhythmia
- Hypertension
- Pneumothorax

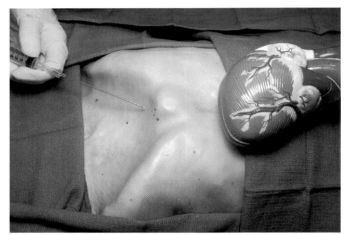

20-1 Needle insertion for pericardiocentesis.

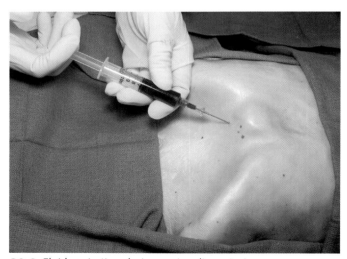

20-2 Fluid aspiration during pericardiocentesis.

POST-PROCEDURE CARE:

1. Monitor vital signs; perform lung and cardiac examinations frequently to assess for complications.

2. Obtain chest x-ray to look for a pneumothorax.

PEARLS/TIPS:

- Needle aspiration should not be performed on patients with a small or loculated effusion.

- Patients with a symptomatic large pericardial effusion and severe decompensation (shock) with tamponade are the ideal candidates for pericardiocentesis. Pericardiocentesis should be performed emergently to achieve hemodynamic stability without waiting for test results.

21. Stress Testing

21a. Treadmill

PURPOSE: To detect the presence or absence of ischemia during exercise. The usual protocols use a gradual increase in speed and elevation of the treadmill.

EQUIPMENT NEEDED:

- Electrocardiogram (ECG) machine

- Treadmill

- Defibrillator

- Crash cart

- Blood pressure cuff

- Cardiopulmonary resuscitation (CPR)-trained personnel present

TECHNIQUE:

1. Record the patient's resting blood pressure and ECG. Leave the blood pressure cuff and ECG leads in place.

2. Start the treadmill at 1.7 miles per hour and have the patient walk while gradually increasing the speed and inclination every 3 minutes (BRUCE protocol).

3. Continue until (a) symptoms develop such as fatigue or chest pain, (b) ECG shows evidence of ischemia with ST depression greater than 1 mm, or (c) ECG shows dysrhythmia.

COMPLICATIONS:

- Dysrhythmia

- Hypotension

- Cardiac arrest

POST-PROCEDURE CARE:

1. Rest patient.

2. Monitor vital signs.

PEARLS/TIPS:

- False positive stress tests are more common in females and may require radioisotope imaging for a better positive predictive value.

- If symptoms of chest pain are present with ST changes, the positive predictive value is better.

- Normal responses include a rise in systolic blood pressure to twice the resting value, with return to baseline 6 minutes after exercise.

- Beta-blockers can mask the heart rate's responses to exercise, so either the patient is asked not to take the beta-blocker on the day of the test, or the presence of beta-blocker is noted on the report.

21b. Pharmacologic

PURPOSE: Evaluate myocardial blood flow to detect ischemia in those who are not candidates for traditional treadmill testing. Dipyridamole, dobutamine, and adenosine increase coronary blood flow, which is lessened in the presence of coronary artery blockage.

EQUIPMENT NEEDED:

- Nuclear medicine capability

- Thallium or technetium (Myoview) cardiac imaging agent

- Dobutamine, dipyridamole, or adenosine

- Crash cart

- Defibrillator

- Blood pressure cuff

- Cardiopulmonary resuscitation (CPR)-trained personnel present
- Intravenous access or Heplock

TECHNIQUE:

1. Inject patient with dobutamine, dipyridamole, or adenosine.

2. Inject patient with thallium or *Myoview* to visualize coronary artery perfusion.

3. Obtain images of the patient's heart in nuclear medicine, and repeat in 4 hours. If there are areas that do not highlight, then the implication is that the thallium or *Myoview* did not reach that area of the heart because of coronary artery blockage.

COMPLICATIONS:

- Dysrhythmia
- Cardiac arrest
- Drug allergies

POST-PROCEDURE CARE:

1. Have the patient rest.

2. Assess vital signs.

PEARLS/TIPS:

- Adenosine has the most rapid onset and shortest half-life.

- Adenosine and dipyridamole can induce bronchospasm, so dobutamine is the drug of choice for patients who have asthma or chronic obstructive pulmonary disease (COPD).

- Beta-blockers may prevent the effect of dobutamine.

22. Venipuncture

PURPOSE: To access a vein for the purpose of withdrawing blood to send to the laboratory for evaluation or placing an indwelling catheter to infuse fluids or medications.

EQUIPMENT NEEDED:

- Tourniquet
- Personal protection equipment (gloves, eye protection, mask, and gown when warranted) for universal precautions
- Alcohol swabs
- Needle appropriate for desired purpose (20-gauge, Vacutainer, or butterfly needle)
- Syringe, 10–30 cc
- Blood specimen tubes
- 2 inch × 2 inch gauze pads
- Self-adhesive bandage
- Labels for patient identification
- Plastic-coated drape

TECHNIQUE:

1. Assemble necessary equipment and position patient appropriately with plastic-coated drape positioned to protect the work area.

2. Apply tourniquet above the antecubital fossa so that it can be quickly removed. The tourniquet should be applied snugly enough so that the venous system will fill but not cause discomfort to the patient. Instruct patient to open and close the fist of the tourniqetted arm to "pump" blood into the superficial venous system.

3. Select the appropriate vein to access by palpating the antecubital fossa for a "full"-feeling vessel. If no adequate vessels are found, assess the ventral aspect of the arm or the dorsal aspect of the hand. Both arms and hands can be assessed to identify the most appropriate vessel to access.

4. Clean the area with the alcohol swab once a vessel is selected.

5. Put on personal protection equipment.

6. Use the nondominant hand to apply traction below the desired site to anchor the vessel.

7. Take the needle in the dominant hand; insert it into the lumen of the vessel with an approach of 15 to 30 degrees to the plane of the arm. If venous blood is not obtained, maintain the needle in its position, repalpate the vessel, and attempt to access the lumen once again.

8. Once the lumen is accessed, withdraw the appropriate amount of blood for the desired tests. Allow blood specimen tube to fill 1/2 to 3/4, then shake the tube once to prevent clotting of the sample.

9. After withdrawing the desired amount of blood, stabilize the needle, remove the tourniquet, place the 2 inch × 2 inch gauze pad over the site, withdraw the needle, and apply direct pressure.

10. Apply the self-adhesive bandage once hemostasis occurs.

11. Fill the blood specimen tubes with appropriate amounts of blood.

12. Label the tubes with the patient's labels and transport to the laboratory.

COMPLICATIONS:

- Pain from tourniquet or venipuncture procedure
- Hematoma at venipuncture site
- Infection at the venipuncture site

POST-PROCEDURE CARE:

1. Check site for hematoma formation.

2. Check for laboratory results.

PEARLS/TIPS:

- Two approaches can be used to access the lumen of the vessel, a direct and an indirect method:

  - Direct: The needle is placed directly over the "full" vessel. As the needle is advanced it passes through the skin and into the lumen of the vein. Using the direct method, the needle may pass through the vessel as it "breaks" through the skin.

  - Indirect: The needle is placed at the lateral edge of the "full" vessel. The needle is first advanced through the skin. After the needle has been advanced under the skin, the vessel can be accessed from the lateral aspect. This approach is beneficial when the patient has tough or leathery skin.

22a. Femoral Venous Access

PURPOSE: The femoral vein can be used when there are no other suitable veins available for access, such as when upper extremity veins cannot be located, or in the presence of swelling or cellulitis. This approach is commonly used in emergency situations when blood samples are urgently needed, for example, during cardiac arrest or trauma resuscitation. One may also consider accessing the femoral vein if the upper extremities have been used for intravenous therapy sites and blood is needed for laboratory evaluation.

EQUIPMENT NEEDED:

- Personal protection equipment (gloves, eye protection, and mask and gown when warranted) for universal precautions

- Alcohol swabs

- Needle appropriate for desired purpose (20-gauge needle 1 1/2 inches long, Vacutainer needle)

- Syringe

- Blood specimen tubes

- 4 inch × 4 inch gauze pads or sponges

- Self-adhesive bandage

- Labels for patient identification

TECHNIQUE:

1. Place the patient in a supine position with the plastic-coated drape protecting the work area.

2. Use the pad of the nondominant index finger to locate the femoral vein by palpating for the pulse of the femoral artery.

3. Cleanse the skin with the alcohol swab by moving in a circular motion from the center out.

4. Palpate for the femoral artery with the nondominant index and middle finger, but make sure not to contaminate the prepared site. (See Figure 14-25.)

5. Insert the needle medial to the femoral artery at an angle perpendicular to the skin. Now position the dominant hand so the syringe's piston can be withdrawn slightly, creating negative pressure in the cylinder (Figure 22-1).

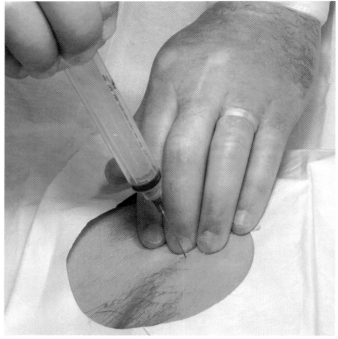

22-1 Needle insertion into femoral vein.

6. Advance the needle slowly toward the femoral vein. Should the vein not be accessed, withdraw the needle slowly but not completely. Advance again toward the position of the femoral vein, angling the needle slightly more medial or lateral but not toward the artery. Repeat this until blood returns into the cylinder of the syringe. Dark blood indicates venous blood (Figure 22-2), whereas bright red blood indicates arterial blood. (Should arterial blood return, proceed with slowly withdrawing the appropriate amount of blood required for laboratory evaluation.)

7. Withdraw the appropriate amount of blood required for laboratory evaluation slowly.

8. Remove the needle quickly once the desired amount of blood is withdrawn, and apply pressure to the puncture site with a 4 inch × 4 inch gauze pad for 5 minutes to ensure hemostasis. Note: If the femoral artery was accessed, greater pressure must be applied for a minimum of 20 minutes after withdrawing the needle to ensure hemostasis. Pressure to the puncture site should be applied by the person performing the procedure, or a designated member of the health care team—*not* by the patient.

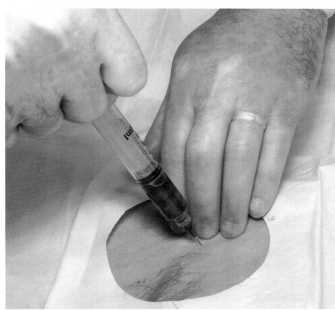

22-2 Venous blood return from femoral vein.

COMPLICATIONS:

- Arterial puncture, laceration, or possibly both can occur.

- Hematoma formation can occur with access of both the femoral vein and artery but is more common if the femoral artery is accessed. This may also occur if appropriate pressure is not applied after withdrawing the needle.

- Discomfort in the leg can occur from femoral nerve irritation during palpation for the femoral artery because of their close proximity.

- Arteriovenous fistulae can form after multiple phlebotomies from the same side.

POST-PROCEDURE CARE:

1. Assess the groin for hematoma formation about 10 to 15 minutes after pressure is released. If you note a hematoma, reapply pressure with a 4 inch × 4 inch gauze for another 15 minutes.

2. Arterial pulses distal to the access site should be assessed.

23. Starting an Intravenous Line

PURPOSE: To gain intravenous access to administer fluids and/or medications.

EQUIPMENT NEEDED (FIGURE 23-1):

- Tourniquet
- Personal protection equipment (gloves, eye protection, and mask and gown when warranted) for universal precautions
- Alcohol swabs
- IV needle (Angiocath) appropriate for desired purpose (18 gauge or greater for hydration or blood administration; 16 gauge or greater for trauma patient resuscitation; 24 gauge or butterfly needle for maintenance fluids or medications)
- Tape (paper or plastic)
- Towel or plastic-coated drape
- Desired IV solution
- IV tubing
- Sterile transparent dressing

TECHNIQUE:

1. Assemble the desired fluid and tubing.

2. Position patient appropriately, and place the towel or plastic-coated drape to protect the work area.

3. Apply the tourniquet above the antecubital fossa so that it can be quickly removed (Figure 23-2). The tourniquet should be applied snugly enough that the venous system will fill but not cause discomfort to the patient. Instruct patient to open and close their fist to "pump" blood into the superficial venous system.

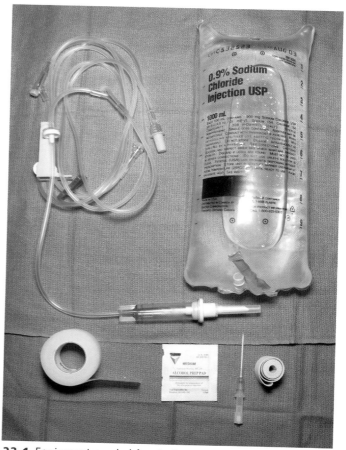

23-1 Equipment needed for starting IV.

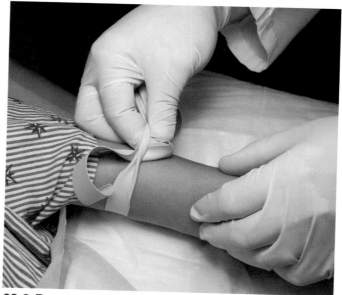

23-2 Tourniquet application.

4. Select the appropriate vein to access by palpating the ventral aspect of the arm for a "full"-feeling vessel. If no adequate vessels are found, assess the dorsal aspect of the hand (Figure 23-3) or the antecubital fossa. Assess both arms and hands to identify the most appropriate vessel to access.

5. Place the plastic-coated drape under the arm to be used once a vessel is selected.

6. Clean the area with the alcohol swab.

7. Use the nondominant hand to apply traction below the desired site to anchor the vessel.

8. Take the needle in the dominant hand; insert it into the lumen of the vessel with an approach of 15 to 30 degrees to the plane of the arm (Figure 23-4). If venous blood is not obtained, maintain the needle in its position, repalpate the vessel, and attempt to access the lumen once again. Once a blood flash is noted in the Angiocath hub, advance the needle or catheter slightly forward to ensure its presence within the lumen (Figure 23-5).

9. Steady the needle with your dominant hand and advance the catheter off the needle with your nondominant hand until the hub of the catheter meets the skin (Figure 23-6).

10. Attach the IV tubing, open the flow controller and assess for flow of fluid. If none is observed, slightly withdraw the catheter and continue to assess for fluid flow. As adequate flow is noted, slowly advance the catheter.

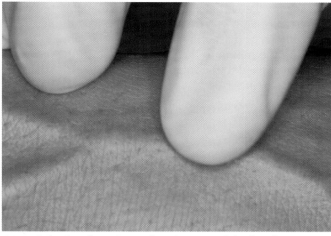

23-3 Palpation for vein on dorsal aspect of the hand.

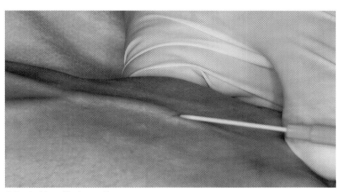

23-4 Needle insertion.

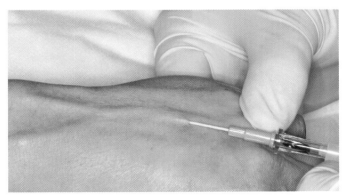

23-5 Advancement of needle.

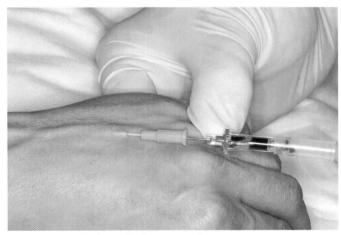

23-6 Removal of needle from IV catheter.

11. Secure the catheter with tape once adequate flow is established by placing a piece around the hub of the catheter and securing it to the skin (Figure 23-7). Secure the tubing to the skin with tape so that any tension applied to the tubing pulls at a site other than the hub's or insertion's.

12. Cover the secured site with the transparent occlusive dressing.

13. Assess the sight for extravasation of IV fluid into surrounding tissue. If the IV fluid does not flow adequately, remove the catheter from the arm, apply pressure for several minutes, then cover with an adhesive bandage, and locate another site (Figure 23-8).

14. Repeat steps 1 to 13 until the IV is successfully established.

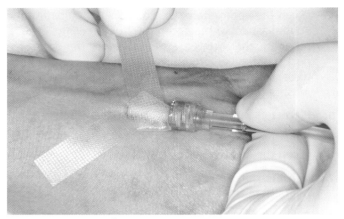

23-7 Securement of IV.

COMPLICATIONS:

- Hematoma formation

- Extravasation of IV fluid

- Phlebitis (chemical and suppurative), cellulitis, bacteremia, and sepsis

POST-PROCEDURE CARE:

1. Instruct the patient to notify health care personnel if they see blood in the IV tubing, if swelling or pain occurs at the IV site, or if IV fluid is not dripping in the chamber.

2. Nursing personnel should assess the IV site daily to ensure that the site is without swelling, redness, or drainage. If signs of infection are not treated, a local infection can lead to bacteremia or sepsis.

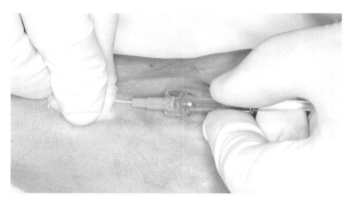

23-8 Removal of IV.

PEARLS/TIPS:

- Valves in the veins may at times inhibit the advancement of the catheter. Should this occur, remove the needle and attach the IV tubing. Initiate a slow flow of fluid and advance the catheter to the hub. Remove the tourniquet from the arm.

- Many inpatient facilities have protocols that require a change in site of IV access every few days to decrease irritation to a vein. This is one opportunity to learn or practice obtaining IV access.

24. Arterial Puncture

 ## 24a. Radial Artery

PURPOSE: To obtain arterial blood for evaluation of acid/base status, oxygenation, and carbon dioxide retention.

EQUIPMENT NEEDED:

- Blood gas sampling kit
- Sterile personal protection equipment (gloves, eye protection, and mask and gown when warranted) for universal precautions
- 5-cc syringe of 1% lidocaine without epinephrine
- Two 25-gauge, 1/2-inch needles
- Plastic bag with ice
- 2 inch × 2 inch gauze pads
- Povidone iodine (Betadine) solution
- Heparin, 10,000 units/mL vial
- Plastic-coated drape
- Washcloth

Note: If a pre-heparinized syringe from a kit is not available, draw 0.5 mL of 10,000 units/mL heparin into a 3-cc plastic syringe. With the tip pointing upward, clear the air, then expel the heparin. There will be enough in the needle to keep the blood from clotting without lowering the pH of the blood.

TECHNIQUE:

1. Perform the Allen's test before radial artery blood sampling:

   a. Have the patient's hand held open with palm facing up.

   b. Palpate both the radial and ulnar arteries.

   c. Instruct the patient to clench the hand tightly.

   d. Occlude both the radial and ulnar arteries by applying direct pressure. Instruct the patient to open the hand; you should observe blanching (pale or white appearance) of the palm.

   e. Release pressure from the ulnar arteries and observe; the pink color should return to the palm within 6 seconds. When this positive result occurs, repeat the preceding steps, releasing pressure from the radial artery this time.

f. Proceed with the procedure if both tests are positive. If the color does not return to the palm within 6 seconds, collateral flow is probably inadequate and the procedure should not be performed on this extremity. Assess the other wrist. Once an adequate vessel is identified, assemble the rest of the equipment.

2. Place the patient's arm on a plastic-coated drape in a relaxed position with the palm facing up.

3. Place a rolled-up washcloth under the wrist, so that it is extended.

4. Use three 2 inch × 2 inch gauze pads soaked in povidone iodine to cleanse the skin over the radial artery. The pads should be used consecutively; start each in the center and clean outward in a circular pattern over the determined puncture site.

5. Put on sterile personal protective equipment.

6. Infiltrate the skin over the planned puncture site with lidocaine.

7. Insert the needle on either side of the artery. Advance it deep into the tissue to the periosteum of the radius. Take care not to aim for the artery. Aspirate to ensure you are not in the vessel.

8. Infiltrate with the lidocaine while withdrawing the needle slowly.

9. Repeat steps 7 and 8 on the opposite side of the artery.

10. Use the nondominant hand in a sterile glove to palpate the radial artery using your index and middle fingers (Figure 24-1). Once you identify the artery, separate your fingers, leaving a space between them.

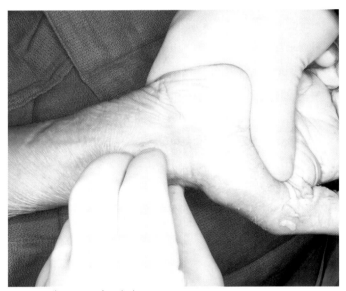

24-1 Palpation of radial artery.

11. Take the syringe from the kit or the 3-cc syringe coated with heparin in your dominant hand. Approaching at an angle of 60 degrees, insert the needle slowly and gently into the skin between your index and middle fingers (Figure 24-2). Advance the needle toward the pulsations palpated by your fingers until bright red blood returns into the syringe. Allow the pressure of the blood to fill the syringe (Figure 24-3).

12. Collect 1 to 2 cc of blood and quickly remove the needle from the skin.

13. Place a 2 inch × 2 inch gauze over the puncture site immediately, and apply pressure for 10 minutes. Simultaneously, position the syringe with the tip upward and tap the side to dislodge any air bubbles, and advance the plunger to express any remaining air.

14. Roll the syringe gently to adequately mix the specimen and prevent clotting.

15. Label the syringe with the appropriate patient identification. Place it in the bag of ice and send to the laboratory.

16. Cover the puncture site with a self-adhesive bandage.

COMPLICATIONS:

- Transient spasm and/or clotting of the radial artery

- Increased risk of arteriovenous fistula or pseudoaneurysm with multiple cannulation attempts of the same artery

- Ischemia and gangrene formation if the arterial supply is compromised. In the case of arterial compromise, a vascular surgeon should be consulted immediately to evaluate the vascular status and treat appropriately.

POST-PROCEDURE CARE:

1. Reassess the puncture site for hematoma formation 15 minutes after pressure has been removed. If you note a hematoma, reapply pressure for another 5 to 10 minutes and reassess.

2. Assess the radial and ulnar arteries for pulsations and the fingernails for capillary refill in less than 2 seconds.

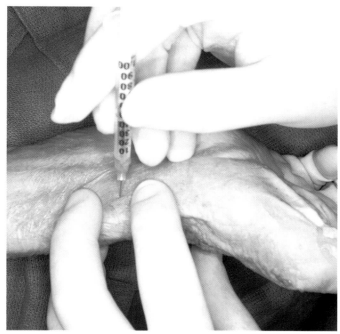

24-2 Needle insertion into radial artery.

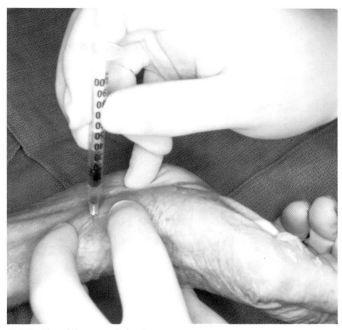

24-3 Blood from radial artery.

PEARLS/TIPS:

- Dominant hand can be rested in the palm of the patient's hand to improve stability and provide ease of approach for the procedure.

- Use of lidocaine is optional. The infiltrated tissue may make identifying the margins of the artery more difficult.

- A negative Allen's test indicates an incomplete superficial palmar arch, which normally includes both the ulnar and radial arteries.

 ## 24b. Femoral Artery

PURPOSE: To obtain arterial blood to assess for acid/base status, oxygenation, and carbon dioxide retention. The femoral artery can be used when there are no other suitable arteries available for access.

EQUIPMENT NEEDED:

- Sterile personal protection equipment (gloves, eye protection, and mask and gown when warranted) to observe universal precautions

- Blood gas sampling kit

- 5-cc syringe with 1% lidocaine without epinephrine

- Two 25-gauge, 1-inch needles

- 4 inch × 4 inch gauze soaked in povidone iodine (Betadine) solution

- Plastic bag with ice

- Heparin, 10,000 units/mL vial

- Sterile drape

- Plastic coated drape

Note: If a pre-heparinized syringe from a kit is not available, draw 0.5 mL of 10,000 units/mL heparin into a 3-cc plastic syringe. With the tip pointing upward, clear the air then expel the heparin. There will be enough in the needle to keep the blood from clotting without lowering the pH of the blood.

TECHNIQUE:

1. Place the patient in a supine position with plastic-coated drape under him or her to protect the work area.

2. Use the pad of your nondominant index finger to palpate for the pulse of the femoral artery (Figure 14-25).

3. Use three 4 inch × 4 inch gauze pads soaked in povidone iodine to cleanse the skin over the femoral artery. The pads should be used consecutively; start each in the center and clean outward in a circular pattern over the designated puncture site.

4. Put on personal protection equipment.

5. Place a fenestrated sterile drape in an appropriate position for the procedure.

6. Infiltrate the skin over the planned puncture site with lidocaine (Figure 14-26).

7. Insert the needle on one side of the artery. Take care not to aim for the artery. Advance the needle deep into the tissue. Aspirate to ensure that you are not in the vessel. Infiltrate with the lidocaine while withdrawing the needle slowly (Figure 24-4).

8. Repeat step 7 on the opposite side of the artery.

9. Use your nondominant hand to palpate the femoral artery with your index and middle fingers. Once you have identified the artery, separate your fingers, leaving a space between them.

10. Take the needle in your dominant hand. Approaching from an angle of 60 degrees, insert the needle slowly and gently into the skin between your index and middle fingers (Figure 24-5).

11. Advance the needle toward the pulsations palpated by your fingers until blood returns into the needle. Allow the pressure of the blood to fill the syringe (Figure 24-6).

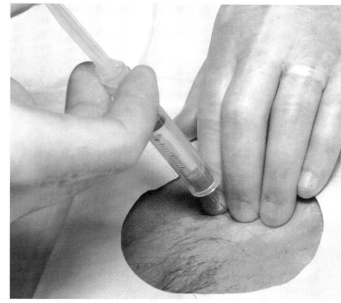

24-4 Deep anesthetization.

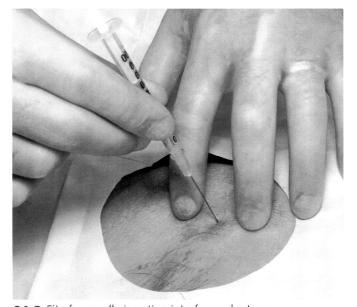

24-5 Site for needle insertion into femoral artery.

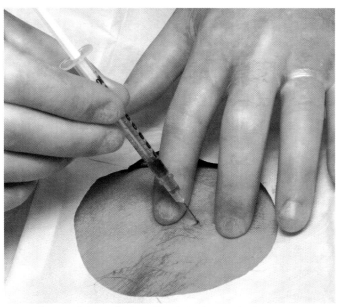

24-6 Successful needle insertion into femoral artery.

12. Collect 1 to 2 cc of blood and quickly remove the needle from the skin.

13. Place a 4 inch $\times$ 4 inch gauze pad over the puncture site immediately and apply pressure for 20 minutes. Simultaneously, position the syringe with the tip upward, tap the side to dislodge any air bubbles, and advance the plunger to express any remaining air.

14. Roll the syringe gently to adequately mix the specimen and prevent clotting.

15. Label the syringe with the appropriate patient identification.

16. Place the specimen in the bag of ice and send it to the laboratory or respiratory therapy department.

17. Cover the puncture site with a self-adhesive bandage.

18. Contact the laboratory or respiratory therapy department for blood gas results.

19. Interpret blood gas results.

COMPLICATIONS:

- Transient spasm and/or clotting of the femoral artery

- Increased risk of arteriovenous fistulae or pseudoaneurysm with multiple cannulation attempts of the same artery

- Embolization of air, clotted blood, or atherosclerotic plaque

- Ischemia and gangrene formation in the foot or toes if the arterial supply is compromised.

- Local hematoma formation, cellulitis, phlebitis, or skin necrosis

- Bacteremia or sepsis

POST-PROCEDURE CARE:

1. Assess the leg, foot, and toes for adequate circulation in 15 minutes. If the artery is compromised, a vascular surgeon should be consulted immediately to evaluate the vascular status and treat appropriately.

PEARLS/TIPS:

- Remember to use the mnemonic "NAVEL" to identify the order of the anatomic structures in the groin. Moving in a lateral-to-medial direction: N = nerve, A = artery, V = vein, E = empty space, L = lymphatics.

25. Arterial Line Placement

25a. Radial Artery

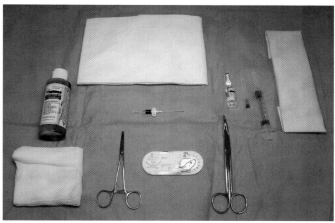

25-1 Equipment for radial artery line placement.

PURPOSE: Allows for constant monitoring of blood pressure when blood pressure cuff measurement is inadequate. Useful when frequent samples of blood are needed for blood gas analysis or other laboratory evaluation.

EQUIPMENT NEEDED (FIGURE 25-1):

- Sterile personal protection equipment (gloves, eye protection, and mask and gown when warranted) to observe universal precautions

- Arm board (long or short)

- Tape (appropriate for patient)

- Rolled washcloth or rolled gauze wrap (Kerlix)

- 4 inch × 4 inch gauze pad soaked in povidone iodine (Betadine)

- Sterile drape

- Plastic-coated drape

- IV catheter (Angiocath) 18- or 20-gauge, 1 1/2 to 2 inches long

- 3-cc syringe fitted with 25-gauge 1-inch needle

- 1% Lidocaine without epinephrine

- Sterile pressure monitoring equipment (tubing, three-way stopcock, heparinized 5% dextrose in water [D5W] equivalent to 1 unit/mL of heparin)

- Monitor with calibrated transducer

- Triple antibiotic ointment

- Sterile occlusive dressing

- Nonabsorbable suture material, size 3-0 on cutting needle

- Suture kit and equipment

TECHNIQUE:

1. Perform an Allen's test before radial artery cannulation (see step 1 of 24a. "Arterial Puncture" for instructions).

2. Assemble the rest of the equipment once an adequate vessel is identified.

3. Place the patient's arm on a plastic-coated drape in a relaxed position with the palm facing up.

4. Place a rolled up washcloth under the wrist, thereby extending it. Secure the arm in this position to the arm board with tape (Figure 25-2).

5. Use three 4 inch × 4 inch gauze pads soaked in povidone iodine to cleanse the skin over the radial artery. The pads should be used consecutively; start each in the center and clean outward in a circular pattern over the determined puncture site.

6. Put on personal protection equipment.

7. Place the fenestrated sterile drape in an appropriate position for the procedure.

8. Infiltrate the skin over the planned puncture site with lidocaine.

9. Insert the needle on one side of the artery. Advance it deep into the tissue to the periosteum of the radius. Take care not to aim for the artery. Aspirate to ensure that you are not in the vessel. Infiltrate with the lidocaine while withdrawing the needle slowly.

10. Repeat step 9 on the opposite side of the artery.

11. Use your nondominant hand in a sterile glove to palpate the radial artery with the index and middle fingers. Once you locate the artery, separate your fingers, leaving a space between them (Figure 25-3).

12. Take the syringe and Angiocath in your dominant hand. Approaching at an angle of 60 degrees, insert the Angiocath slowly and gently into the skin between your index and middle fingers (Figure 25-4).

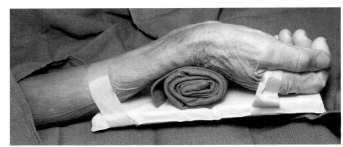

25-2 Hand secured to arm board.

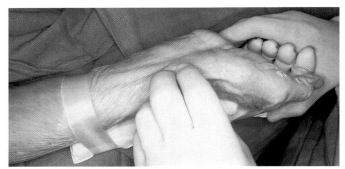

25-3 Palpation of radial artery.

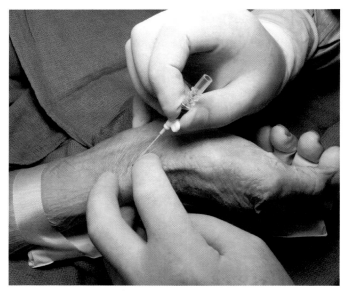

25-4 Insertion point for IV catheter.

13. Advance the needle toward the pulse that you palpated with your fingers until blood returns into the Angiocath hub (Figure 25-5). If the Angiocath advances to the periosteum without blood return, slowly withdraw the Angiocath without removing it, in case it has passed through the artery.

14. Redirect the needle tip toward the arterial pulse, and advance it slowly if you obtain no blood return. Repeat as needed.

15. Advance the Angiocath 2 to 3 mm more when you get blood return; stabilize the needle hub, then advance the catheter off the needle into the arterial lumen (Figure 25-6).

16. Apply pressure distal to the catheter tip to restrict the backflow of blood.

17. Remove the needle.

18. Attach sterile pressure tubing.

19. Flush the catheter.

20. Assess monitor for adequate wave form.

21. Reposition catheter to obtain an adequate wave form. (If you are unable to establish adequate waveform, remove the catheter. Apply pressure to insertion site for 10 minutes to obtain hemostasis.)

22. Secure the hub of the catheter with nonabsorbable suture (Figure 25-7).

23. Apply triple antibiotic ointment at the insertion site.

24. Cover the ointment and site with sterile transparent occlusive dressing.

25. Attempt to establish an arterial line at another site by repeating previous steps.

COMPLICATIONS:

- Transient spasm and/or clotting of the radial artery

- Increased risk of arteriovenous fistulae or pseudoaneurysm with multiple cannulation attempts of the same artery

- Embolization of air, clotted blood, or atherosclerotic plaque

- Ischemia and gangrene formation in the hand/fingers if the arterial supply is compromised

- Local hematoma formation, cellulitis, phlebitis, or skin necrosis

- Bacteremia and sepsis

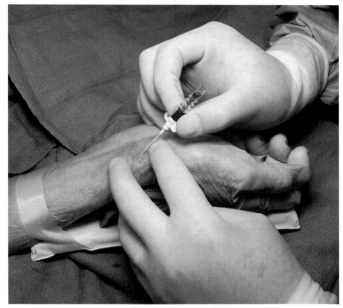

25-5 Insertion of IV catheter into radial artery.

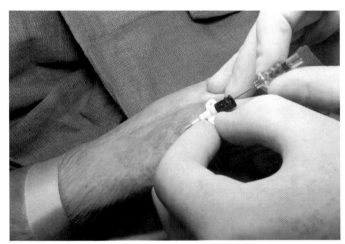

25-6 Removal of needle from IV catheter.

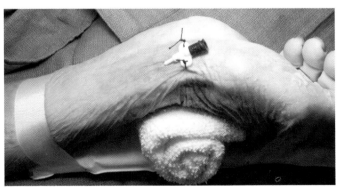

25-7 Securement of IV catheter.

POST-PROCEDURE CARE:

1. Assess the hand and fingers for adequate circulation. If the artery is compromised, a vascular surgeon should be consulted immediately to evaluate the vascular status and treat appropriately.

2. Assess the site daily for cellulitis and change dressing at appropriate intervals.

3. Remove the catheter as soon as the patient's condition stabilizes and frequent blood sampling is no longer needed. This will limit the possibility of local cellulitis, bacteremia, or sepsis.

PEARLS/TIPS:

- Your dominant hand can rest in the palm of the patient's hand to improve stability and provide ease of approach for the procedure.

- Use of lidocaine is optional. The infiltrated tissue may make identifying the margins of the artery more difficult.

25b. Femoral Artery

PURPOSE: The femoral artery can be used when there are no other suitable arteries available for access.

EQUIPMENT NEEDED (FIGURE 25-8):

- Sterile personal protection equipment (gloves, eye protection, and mask and gown when warranted) for universal precautions

- Paper or plastic tape (as appropriate for patient)

- 4 inch × 4 inch gauze pads soaked in povidone iodine (Betadine)

- Sterile fenestrated drape

- Plastic-coated drape

- IV catheter (Angiocath) 18-gauge, 4 to 6 inches long

- 5-cc syringe with 25-gauge 1 1/2-inch needle

- 1% Lidocaine without epinephrine

- Sterile pressure monitoring equipment (tubing, three-way stopcock, heparinized 5% dextrose in water [D5W] solution equivalent to 1 unit/mL of heparin)

- Monitor with calibrated transducer

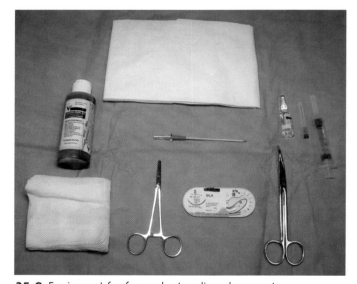

25-8 Equipment for femoral artery line placement.

- Triple antibiotic ointment

- Sterile occlusive dressing

- Nonabsorbable suture material, size 3-0 on cutting needle

- Suture kit and equipment

TECHNIQUE:

1. Place the patient in a supine position with the plastic-coated drape protecting the work area.

2. Use the pad of your nondominant index finger to palpate for the pulse of the femoral artery (Figure 14-25).

3. Use three 4 inch × 4 inch gauze pads soaked in povidone iodine to cleanse the skin over the femoral artery. The pads should be used consecutively; start each in the center and clean outward in a circular pattern over the determined puncture site.

4. Put on sterile personal protection equipment.

5. Place a fenestrated sterile drape in an appropriate position for the procedure.

6. Infiltrate the skin over the planned puncture site with lidocaine without epinephrine (see Figure 14-26).

7. Insert the needle on one side of the artery. Take caution not to aim for the artery. Advance the needle deep into the tissue (see Figure 24-4).

8. Aspirate to ensure that you are not in the vessel.

9. Infiltrate with the lidocaine while withdrawing the needle slowly.

10. Repeat steps 7 and 8 on the opposite side of the artery.

11. Use your nondominant hand to palpate the femoral artery using the index and middle fingers. Once identified, separate your fingers, leaving a space between them.

12. Take the Angiocath in the dominant hand. Approaching at an angle of 60 degrees, insert the needle slowly and gently into the skin between your index and middle fingers (Figure 25-9).

13. Advance the needle toward the pulse you have palpated with your fingers until blood returns into the hub of the Angiocath. If you do not access the artery, withdraw the needle slowly but not completely. Advance again toward the position of the femoral artery. Repeat this until blood returns into the hub of the needle (Figure 25-10).

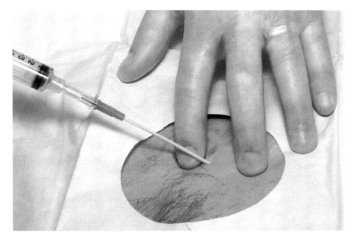

25-9 Insertion of IV catheter, approaching at a 60° angle.

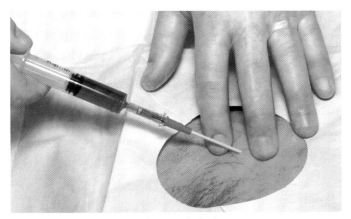

25-10 Blood return into the needle hub.

14. Advance the Angiocath slightly farther once blood return is obtained, then stabilize the needle hub and advance the catheter off the needle into the arterial lumen.

15. Stabilize the catheter, then quickly withdraw the needle and attach the pressure monitor tubing (Figures 25-11 and 25-12).

16. Flush the catheter with saline or heparin.

17. Assess monitor for adequate wave form. (If you are unable to establish adequate waveform, remove the catheter. Apply pressure to insertion site for 10 minutes to obtain hemostasis.)

18. Reposition the catheter to obtain adequate wave form.

19. Secure the hub of catheter with nonabsorbable suture (Figure 25-13).

20. Apply triple antibiotic ointment at site.

21. Cover with sterile transparent occlusive dressing.

22. Attempt to establish arterial line at another site by repeating previous steps.

COMPLICATIONS:

- Transient spasm and/or clotting of the femoral artery

- Increased risk of arteriovenous fistula or pseudoaneurysm with multiple cannulation attempts of the same artery

- Embolization of air, clotted blood, or atherosclerotic plaque

- Ischemia and gangrene formation in the leg, foot, or toes if the arterial supply is compromised

- Local hematoma formation, cellulitis, phlebitis, or skin necrosis

- Bacteremia or sepsis

POST-PROCEDURE CARE:

1. Assess the leg, foot, and toes for adequate circulation every few hours. In the event of arterial compromise, consult a vascular surgeon immediately to evaluate the vascular status and treat appropriately.

2. Assess the site daily for cellulitis, and change dressing at appropriate intervals.

3. Remove the catheter as soon as the patient's condition stabilizes and frequent blood sampling is no longer needed. This will limit the possibility of local cellulitis, bacteremia, or sepsis.

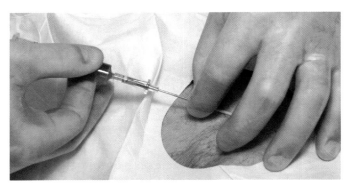

25-11 Removal of needle from catheter.

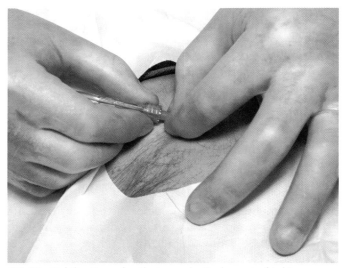

25-12 Stabilization of catheter and attachment of tubing.

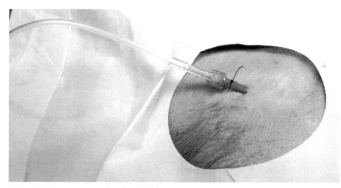

25-13 Securement of catheter.

- Remember to use the mnemonic "NAVEL" to identify the order of the anatomical structures in the groin. Moving from a lateral to medial direction: N = nerve, A = artery, V = vein, E = empty space, L = lymphatics.

26. Blood Pressure Measurement

PURPOSE: To assess the patient's blood pressure.

EQUIPMENT NEEDED:

- Stethoscope
- Blood pressure cuff (sphygmomanometer)

TECHNIQUE:

1. Measure blood pressure with patient seated and his or her arm resting on a table.

2. Position the patient's arm so that it is slightly flexed at the same level as the patient's heart, if possible. The patient's upper arm should be bare. Avoid constricting the upper arm if the sleeve must be rolled up, or the subsequent BP reading will be falsely elevated.

3. Wrap the blood pressure cuff snugly around the patient's upper arm, positioning it so that the lower edge of the cuff is 1 inch above the antecubital fossa.

4. Locate the brachial artery on the medial aspect of the elbow by palpating for the pulse, then place the stethoscope over this point, below the cuff (Figure 26-1). Avoid rubbing the stethoscope on the cuff or any clothing, because these noises may block out the pulse sounds.

5. Close the valve on the rubber inflating bulb and squeeze it rapidly to inflate the cuff until the dial or column of mercury reads 30 mm Hg higher than the usual systolic pressure. If the usual systolic pressure is unknown, inflate the cuff to 210 mm Hg.

6. Open the valve slightly, allowing the pressure to fall gradually (2 to 3 mm Hg per second). As the pressure falls, record the level on the dial or mercury tube at which the pulsing is first heard. This is the systolic pressure.

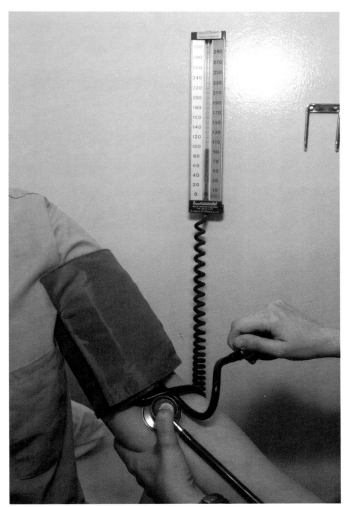

26-1 Proper placement of stethoscope and blood pressure cuff.

7. Listen as the air continues to be let out, as the sounds will fade. Record the point at which the sound completely disappears. This is the diastolic pressure.

COMPLICATIONS:

• Discomfort from the blood pressure cuff

POST-PROCEDURE CARE:

1. Instruct the patient to return for further evaluation if the blood pressure reading was high (at the provider's discretion).

PEARLS/TIPS:

• Correct positioning of the stethoscope is important to get an accurate recording.

26a. Orthostatic Blood Pressure (Tilt Test)

PURPOSE: To assess the vascular, fluid volume, or hydration status of a patient.

EQUIPMENT NEEDED:

• Blood pressure cuff (sphygmomanometer)

• Stethoscope

TECHNIQUE:

1. Place the patient in the supine position.

2. Place the blood pressure cuff on the patient's upper arm. Ensure that you are using an appropriate-sized blood pressure cuff for the patient's size. The blood pressure cuff should fit comfortably around the patient's arm and remain in place during the procedure.

3. Take the patient's blood pressure and record it.

4. Take the patient's pulse and record it.

5. Place the patient in the sitting position and wait 2 minutes to allow the blood pressure and pulse to equilibrate to the new position, thus obtaining a more accurate measurement.

6. Repeat steps 3 and 4.

7. Place the patient in the standing position and wait 2 minutes to allow the blood pressure and pulse to equilibrate to the new position. **Note:** Remain close to the patient in case he or she becomes faint or collapses. This will allow you to assist the patient back to bed safely or to guide them to the floor.

8. Repeat steps 3 and 4.

9. Compare the readings. Look for one of the following. One or both of these changes suggests that the patient's body cannot compensate for drastic positional changes, because of dehydration, hypovolemia, or acute anemia.

   a. A decrease in the blood pressure by 10 or more mm Hg from the lying to sitting positions or from the sitting to standing positions.

   b. Increase in the pulse rate by 10 or more beats per minute from the lying to sitting positions or from the sitting to standing positions.

10. Institute appropriate treatment immediately. Continue monitoring until symptoms resolve.

COMPLICATIONS:

• Discomfort from the blood pressure cuff

• Injury secondary to collapse from performing procedure

POST-PROCEDURE CARE:

1. Repeat the procedure daily until symptoms resolve.

PEARLS/TIPS:

• The pulse should be taken immediately after monitoring the blood pressure.

• An electronic blood pressure monitor can be used to get a simultaneous blood pressure and pulse rate.

• Patients need close monitoring while performing the procedure to ensure their safety if they fall.

27. Doppler Blood Pressure

PURPOSE: To evaluate the patient's blood pressure when it cannot be obtained by either standard blood pressure measurement or palpated blood pressure.

EQUIPMENT NEEDED:

- Blood pressure cuff (sphygmomanometer)
- Doppler ultrasonography device
- Medium for doppler (KY jelly, ultrasound gel)

TECHNIQUE:

1. Place patient in the supine position.

2. Place the blood pressure cuff on the patient's upper arm. Ensure that you are using an appropriate-sized blood pressure cuff for the patient's size.

3. Apply doppler medium over the patient's brachial or radial artery.

4. Turn on the doppler and place the transducer over the brachial or radial artery, and position the transducer tip so that you can hear the maximal pulse.

5. Inflate the blood pressure cuff slowly until you can no longer hear the pulsations, and continue to inflate the cuff to a pressure of 15 mm Hg greater than that level.

6. Deflate the cuff slowly.

7. Note the pressure reading when you hear the pulsations again.

8. Repeat the procedure to ensure an accurate reading.

9. Ensure that appropriate treatment is administered.

COMPLICATIONS:

- Discomfort from the use of the blood pressure cuff

POST-PROCEDURE CARE:

1. Continue to use this method until blood pressure improves, enabling the use of standard monitoring methods.

2. Consider use of central arterial monitoring if blood pressure does not improve or worsens with appropriate medical treatment.

3. Arrange consultation with appropriate specialist if you suspect vascular compromise.

28. Blood Culture

PURPOSE: To determine whether organisms are present in the blood of a patient suspected of being bacteremic or septic.

EQUIPMENT NEEDED:

- Tourniquet
- Personal protection equipment (gloves, eye protection, and mask and gown when warranted) for universal precautions
- 4 inch × 4 inch gauze pads or swabs, one set soaked in alcohol and the other soaked in povidone iodine (Betadine) solution.
- Syringe, 20 mL or Vacutainer set
- Needle, 20-gauge, 1 to 1 1/2 inches, or Vacutainer needle
- Sterile gauze pads, 4 inch × 4 inch
- Blood culture bottles (Figure 28-1)
- Self-adhesive bandage
- Labels with patient identification

TECHNIQUE:

1. Select a venipuncture site. Avoid femoral veins and contaminated sites (such as areas near skin breakdown). Do not draw cultures from an indwelling intravenous catheter.

2. Place a tourniquet proximal to desired site.

3. Prepare venipuncture site antiseptically. Use three swabs sequentially, each soaked in povidone iodine; wipe in a circular motion from the center out to about 6 to 8 cm. Let the povidone iodine solution dry on the skin for 2 minutes.

4. Put on personal protection equipment.

5. Wipe the site clean of povidone iodine in a sterile fashion with an alcohol swab. Let the alcohol dry.

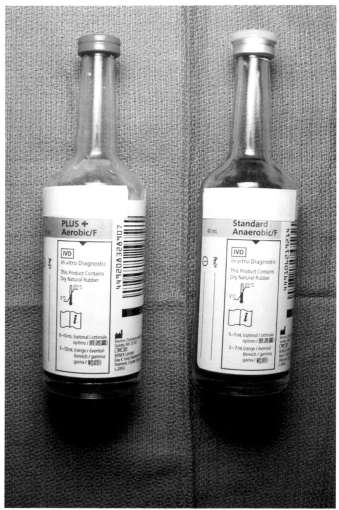

28-1 Blood culture bottles.

6. Perform the venipuncture without palpating the puncture site, so as not to contaminate the site (see 22. "Venipuncture" for instructions).

7. Draw blood into the syringe. Withdraw approximately 10 to 15 mL for an adult and 2 to 5 mL for a child.

8. Release the tourniquet; quickly withdraw the needle, maintaining sterile technique. Immediately place a 4 inch × 4 inch sterile gauze pad over the site. Apply pressure for hemostasis.

9. Clean the top of the blood culture bottle with alcohol or povidone iodine.

10. Pierce the rubber stopper on top of the bottle with the needle and allow the vacuum to draw the blood into the bottle. *Do not remove the cap from the top under any circumstances,* because this would result in an aerobic instead of an anaerobic culture and thus compromise the accuracy of the test.

11. Label the bottle with the appropriate information immediately, place in the appropriate transport container and send it to the microbiology lab.

COMPLICATIONS:

- Pain from tourniquet or venipuncture procedure
- Hematoma at venipuncture site
- Infection at the venipuncture site

POST-PROCEDURE CARE:

1. Check the site for hematoma formation.

2. Check for culture results at 24 and 48 hours from blood draw and continue to follow as needed.

PEARLS/TIPS:

- Ensure that site is adequate before prepping with povidone iodine.
- Allowing the povidone iodine to dry decreases the risk of culture contamination.

29. Glucose Monitoring

PURPOSE: To assess a patient's blood glucose level.

EQUIPMENT NEEDED:

- Glucometer
- Finger lancet

TECHNIQUE:

1. Calibrate the glucometer by following its instructions.

2. Obtain a finger stick sample of blood from the patient using the lancet.

3. Place the sample of blood on a test strip. Insert the test strip into the glucometer. After about 30 seconds, the measurement of the *capillary* blood glucose is displayed on the monitor.

4. Instruct the patient to self-administer insulin on a sliding scale as needed to improve the control of their diabetes.

COMPLICATIONS:

- Persistent bleeding if the patient is on anticoagulant therapy (very rare)

POST-PROCEDURE CARE:

1. Frequency of monitoring is up to the individual physician and patient. The best times are: during fasting; 30 minutes preprandial; and 2 hours postprandial. It can take 2 hours for regular insulin to take effect, so when the patient self-administers insulin, it is best to have them recheck their blood sugar in 2 hours.

PEARLS/TIPS:

- Glucometers use a capillary sample instead of the standard venous sample, so there is a standard degree of inaccuracy in every machine, and the actual numbers are available on the product information for each glucometer.

- The glucometer has a system of calibration to optimize its function. The machine must be calibrated at least daily; also it should be calibrated every time a new box of test strips is opened.

- Continuous glucose monitoring:

  - Portable insulin infusion device.

  - Insulin is delivered through an indwelling 25-gauge scalp vein needle that is positioned under the skin and connected to the insulin pump by a catheter. The needle site is changed every other day to avoid infection and blockage of the needle itself.

  - Insulin is infused at a constant basal rate of 0.5 to 2.0 units/hour. The infusion device can be programmed for up to four different basal rates within a 24-hour period. A bolus is delivered before each meal.

VI. Abdomen

30. Paracentesis

PURPOSE: To diagnose certain disease processes on the basis of ascitic fluid composition, and to provide a therapeutic intervention by removing excess fluid from the abdominal cavity.

EQUIPMENT NEEDED (FIGURE 30-1):

- Skin cleanser such as povidone iodine (Betadine)
- 1% Lidocaine
- Sterile gloves and mask
- Sterile marking pen
- Sterile drapes and towels
- Syringes (5 cc and 20 cc)
- Needles (22- and 25-gauge)
- Three-way stopcock
- IV tubing
- IV catheter (20 gauge for therapeutic purposes, 18 gauge for diagnosis)
- 500 to 1000 mL vacuum bottle and IV drip set (therapeutic)

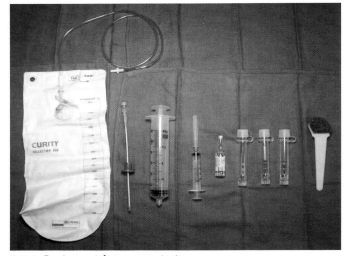

30-1 Equipment for paracentesis.

TECHNIQUE:

1. Check the patient's prothrombin time/partial thromboplastin time (PT/PTT) before this procedure to prepare for any bleeding complications.

2. Ask the patient to empty his or her bladder before the procedure; arrange the patient in a supine position.

3. Use physical exam techniques (e.g., percussion, shifting dullness) to determine the presence of ascites.

4. Clean the skin with cleansing solution, typically Betadine. Cleanse the area using sterile gauze that has been soaked in the cleaning solution. Clean the area in a circular motion moving from the center outward. This should be repeated for a minimum of three times.

5. Place the sterile drapes around the area to be tapped.

6. Mark the entry site at or just below the umbilicus, the lower quadrant (anterior iliac spine), or lateral to the rectus muscle if there is a scar or bowel sounds present on physical examination.

7. Infiltrate the skin and subcutaneous tissue with lidocaine using the 25-gauge needle and a 5-cc syringe (Figure 30-2).

8. Use the 22-gauge needle and 20-cc syringe, and direct the needle at a perpendicular/oblique angle to the skin aiming toward the pelvic hollow and applying slight suction to the syringe as you slowly advance (Figure 30-3).

9. *Stop* advancing the needle as soon as ascitic fluid enters the syringe. Keep the needle in place and remove only the syringe. Send the fluid off for studies (Figure 30-4). This is a diagnostic tap. See step 11 for removal of the needle.

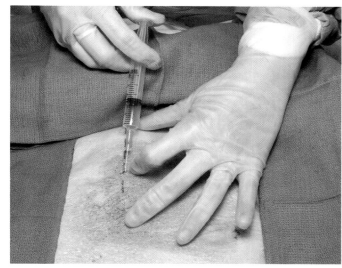

30-2 Anesthetizing skin for paracentesis procedure.

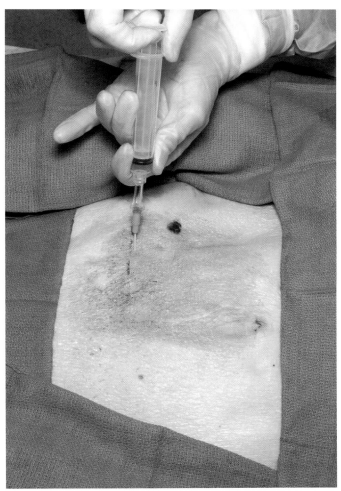

30-3 Needle insertion for paracentesis.

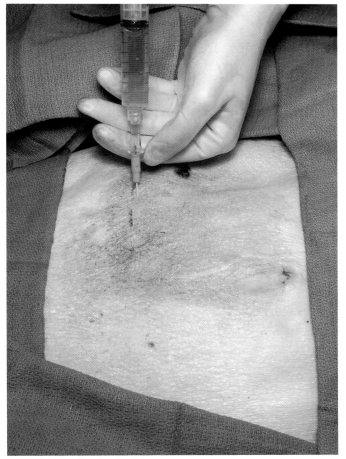

30-4 Ascitic fluid collection.

10. For a therapeutic tap, attach the IV tubing to the 22-gauge needle, the end of which is attached to the bottle, and allow the fluid to drain. The tubing should have a three-way stopcock attached to control the amount of fluid that enters the bottles. It is important to drain off no more than 1 liter at a time in a therapeutic tap, to allow the body to compensate for the sudden shift in fluid.

11. Remove the needle in a "Z" pattern as you retract it from the skin; this minimizes the chance of an ongoing leakage of ascitic fluid.

COMPLICATIONS:

- Hypotension
- Perforation of the bowel
- Hemorrhage
- Infection
- Persistent ascitic leak
- Bladder perforation

POST-PROCEDURE CARE:

1. Watch for hypotension immediately post-procedure. This complication can be avoided somewhat by hydrating the patient during the procedure with IV fluids or by replacing a small amount of albumin for each liter removed.

PEARLS/TIPS:

- Always advance the needle slowly to prevent trauma to the internal organs. If you are unable successfully to perform the paracentesis at the bedside, consult radiology for an ultrasound-guided tap.

- The most commonly ordered labs for ascitic fluid include glucose, protein, amylase, triglycerides, cell count, cytology, Gram stain or culture, and pH.

VII. Back

31. Lumbar Puncture

PURPOSE: To diagnose central nervous system infections, subarachnoid hemorrhages, and many other neurologic pathologies.

EQUIPMENT NEEDED (FIGURE 31-1):

- Spinal or lumbar puncture tray (specifically the items listed below)
- Sterile gloves
- Manometer
- Three-way stopcock
- Sterile dressing
- Antiseptic solution with skin swabs
- Sterile drape
- 1% Lidocaine
- 3-cc syringe
- 20- and 25-gauge needle
- 20- and 22-gauge spinal needle
- Four plastic test tubes, numbered 1 to 4, with caps

TECHNIQUE:

1. Obtain informed consent from the patient or next of kin.

2. Obtain a CT scan of the head or perform a fundoscopic exam to check for papilledema. It is absolutely necessary to rule out increased intracranial pressure before proceeding.

3. Place the patient in a sitting position on the edge of the bed (much like the position for a spinal or epidural) or in a lateral recumbent position (lying on the side with knees tucked to chest and chin to chest) (Figure 31-2).

4. Locate the L3-L4 space. To do this, find the iliac crests and move your fingers medially from the crests to the spine.

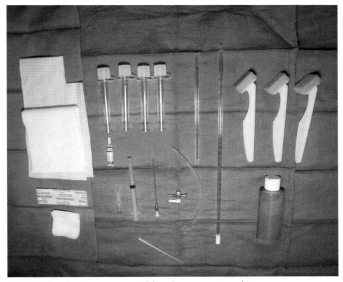

31-1 Standard commercial lumbar puncture kit.

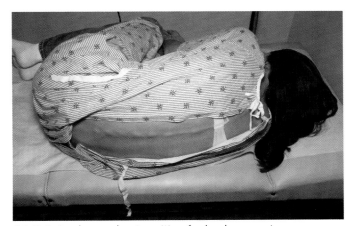

31-2 Lateral recumbent position for lumbar puncture.

5. Mark the entry site with your thumbnail or a marker (Figure 31-3).

6. Open and prepare the spinal tray in a sterile manner.

7. Assemble the stopcock on the manometer and set it aside, ensuring that everything is kept sterile.

8. Use the skin swabs and sterile antiseptic solution to clean the skin at the interspace you have chosen, along with the space below (in case you need to move to the lower space after a failed attempt). Clean the L3-L4 space in a circular fashion starting at the center and moving outward. (Do not spill cleaning solution on the tray.)

9. Place the sterile drape on the patient.

10. Use the 25-gauge needle and the 3-cc syringe to administer the 1% lidocaine intradermally, creating a skin wheal.

11. Remove the 25-gauge needle, and use the 20-gauge needle to anesthetize the deeper subcutaneous tissue.

12. Open the plastic numbered test tubes and place them upright in the preformed circular slots in the tray while you are waiting for the lidocaine to take effect.

13. Insert the spinal needle (20- or 22-gauge) through the skin wheal between the L3 and L4 spinous processes at a slightly cephalad angle toward the umbilicus (Figure 31-4).

14. Advance the needle slowly but smoothly. Usually a characteristic "pop" is felt as the needle passes through the dura (usually 4 to 5 cm into the skin).

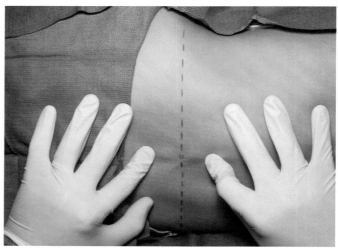

31-3 Lumbar puncture landmarks.

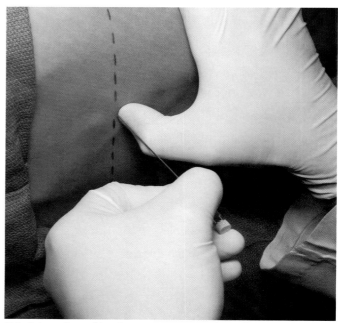

31-4 Insertion of lumbar puncture spinal needle.

15. Stop and remove the stylus to observe for fluid return once you think you have felt the pop (Figure 31-5). If you see no fluid, you have not yet passed through the dura and you must replace the stylus and advance a few millimeters to recheck.

16. Attach the stopcock to the needle once cerebrospinal fluid (CSF) is seen in the needle hub, and turn the stopcock to allow flow into the manometer. This is the opening pressure. Make a mental note of the pressure and color of the CSF.

17. Switch the stopcock to collect about 3 cc of CSF in the four plastic numbered tubes starting with tube number 1 (Figure 31-6).

18. Remove the needle from the patient's back.

19. Place a sterile dressing on the site and have the patient stay in the supine position for 2 hours.

COMPLICATIONS:

- Post-spinal puncture headache
- Brain herniation
- Bloody tap (may lead to hematoma)
- Meningitis

POST-PROCEDURE CARE:

1. Send the four tubes for the following labs:

   a. Tube 1, bacteriology: Gram stain, culture and sensitivity, acid-fast bacilli, fungal cultures and stains, cell count (compare with tube 3 to differentiate traumatic tap from subarachnoid hemorrhage).

   b. Tube 2, biochemistry: glucose, protein, and electrophoresis (if working up for multiple sclerosis to detect oligoclonal banding).

   c. Tube 3, hematology: cell count with differential.

   d. Tube 4, special studies if needed: VDRL (neurosyphilis), India ink (*Cryptococcus neoformans*).

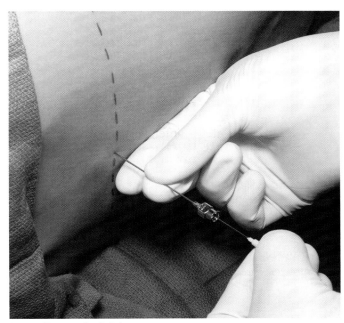

31-5 Removal of stylus.

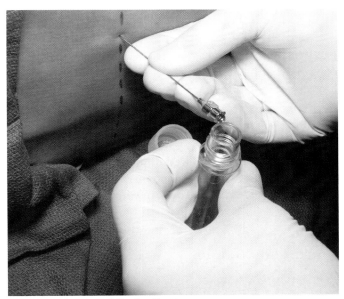

31-6 Cerebrospinal fluid collection.

- Contraindications include:
    - ◆ Puncture site infection
    - ◆ Anticoagulation
    - ◆ Increased intracranial pressure
    - ◆ Thrombocytopenia
- Remember that the spinal cord ends at the conus medullaris, which is at about the L2 level in adults.
- The smaller the needle used for lumbar puncture, the smaller the risk of post-spinal puncture headache.
- To prevent herniation, make sure patient does not have increased intracranial pressure (no papilledema, or a negative CT).

32. Epidural and Spinal Block

PURPOSE: To achieve analgesia for postoperative pain control, labor pains, lower abdominal or pelvic surgery, or lower extremity surgery.

EQUIPMENT NEEDED:

- Epidural tray or spinal tray should contain sterile gauze, sterile cleaning solution (such as povidone iodine), three cleaning sponges, sterile saline (0.9% NaCl), glass syringe, 18-gauge epidural needle, epidural catheter
- 1-cc syringe
- Extra filter needle
- Fentanyl or sufentanil
- Two pairs of sterile gloves
- 25-gauge spinal needle
- 1% Lidocaine
- 1.5% Lidocaine with epinephrine
- Tape
- Clear semipermeable adhesive film (Opsite)
- 0.75% Bupivacaine
- 0.02 cc (10 μg sufentanil)
- Assistant

TECHNIQUE #1—EPIDURAL CATHETER INSERTION:

1. Obtain informed consent from the patient or next of kin.

2. Have the patient sit on the side of the bed with his or her feet comfortably on a stool or chair (Figure 32-1). At times the patient will be unable to sit comfortably on the side of the bed; at this point it may be warranted to perform the procedure with the patient in the lateral decubitus position. Coach the patient on proper position.

3. Stand behind the patient and verbally communicate each step of the process.

4. Locate the posterior iliac crests and then the L4 vertebra by moving fingers from crests horizontally toward midline (Figure 32-1).

5. Palpate the L4 vertebra, then move superiorly off the spinous process and into the space between L3 and L4. The space must be well delineated.

6. Press a firm, visible mark in the skin using your thumb nail.

7. Put on sterile gloves, and open the epidural or spinal tray (make sure to keep tray sterile).

8. Have an assistant drop the extra 1-cc syringe and the extra filter needle onto the tray in a sterile fashion.

9. Open package of sterile cleaning solution and pour into receptacle.

10. Clean the L3-L4 space in a circular fashion with the three supplied cleaning sponges. (Do not spill cleaning solution on the epidural or spinal tray.)

11. Arrange the sterile drape (you may need your assistant to apply some tape to firmly secure the drape).

12. Dry the L3-L4 space with supplied sterile gauze. If the above is done in a timely fashion, your thumbnail mark should still be visible. If not, repalpate the L3-L4 space.

13. Anesthetize the skin by making a skin wheal with the 1% lidocaine in a 3-cc syringe and 25-gauge needle.

14. Anesthetize deeper tissue through the skin wheal.

15. Prepare epidural tray while waiting for skin analgesia.

16. Open the vial of 1.5% lidocaine with epinephrine.

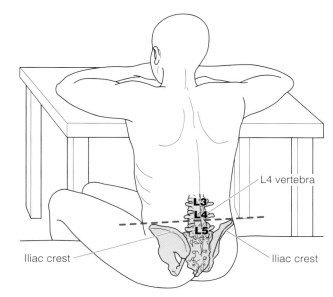

32-1 Proper epidural position and location of L4 vertebra.

17. Draw 3 cc through filter and place this "test dose" to the side. Prepare the supplied glass syringe by lubricating the interior with the supplied sterile saline through filter. Some prefer to have 2 cc of saline with a small bubble inside the glass syringe, while others remove all fluid and use only air. Regardless, have the glass syringe pulled back 2 to 3 cc and ready to attach to 18-gauge epidural needle when needed. Skin analgesia should have been obtained by now.

18. Insert 18-gauge epidural needle with bevel upward through skin wheal into the interspinous ligament.

19. Attach glass syringe with 2 to 3 cc of air or saline.

20. Advance epidural needle slowly.

21. Keep needle stabilized with the nondominant hand by resting dorsal surface of hand on patient's back. Most epidural needles have markings in centimeters.

22. Advance needle slowly while pulsating the glass syringe. While in the ligament, a firm resistance should be felt with each pulsation of the glass syringe.

23. Advance needle slowly. Most epidural spaces will be found at a depth of 4 to 6 cm. Once the needle enters the epidural space, resistance to thumb pulsations will markedly decrease.

24. Remove glass syringe and watch for cerebrospinal fluid (CSF) return. If no CSF returns, continue procedure and place epidural catheter through epidural needle. Catheter should be inserted 5 to 6 cm into epidural space (so if the 18-gauge needle is 5 cm at the skin, the catheter should be inserted to 10 cm at the skin). Never withdraw the catheter back through the needle, because this could sever the catheter.

25. Remove 18-gauge epidural needle (*do not* remove catheter with needle).

26. Insert exposed end of catheter into catheter adapter and snap the wings of the adapter together.

27. Administer "test dose" of 3 cc 1.5% lidocaine with epinephrine. Remember to aspirate first. A negative aspiration is one in which no blood is aspirated back though catheter.

28. Observe patient's heart rate and ask patient if he or she experiences any symptoms of intravascular injection such as ringing in the ears or a metallic taste.

29. After intravascular placement of catheter is ruled out, place an adhesive-backed catheter pad and secure catheter to patient's back with clear Opsite and tape.

30. Remove sterile drape and place patient back into supine position. You have completed the procedure and are now ready to connect the epidural catheter to an infusion pump if so desired.

TECHNIQUE #2—SPINAL BLOCK:

1. Prepare patient as above in steps 1 through 14.

2. Draw up the medication desired for spinal block while waiting for skin analgesia. A dose of 1.6 cc of 0.75% bupivacaine and 0.2 cc (10 μg) of sufentanil will suffice for an adult of average height. Remember to use a filter needle. Instead of the 18-gauge epidural needle, use the included sterile introducer needle and the 24-gauge spinal needle.

3. Place the introducer through the skin wheal into the interspinous ligament.

4. Place spinal needle into the introducer needle and slowly advance. You should feel a characteristic "pop" and loss of resistance when the dura has been punctured.

5. Remove the stylet from the spinal needle and observe CSF return.

6. Connect the spinal needle with the syringe of local anesthetic and opioid.

7. Aspirate and observe the CSF form a swirl in syringe.

8. Administer the medication, and remove all needles from the patient's back.

9. Place the patient in a supine position and check the anesthesia "level" with an alcohol pad and/or sharp plastic needle. A level of about T6-T4 (about nipple line) is adequate for most procedures.

COMPLICATIONS:

- Epidural
  - Hypotension
  - Unintentional dural puncture (wet tap)
  - Intravascular catheter insertion
- Spinal block
  - Unexpected high block

POST-PROCEDURE CARE:

1. All patients who have had an epidural should be seen 24 hours after catheter removal to ensure intact sensation and motor function.

PEARLS/TIPS:

- Contraindications:
  - Patient refusal
  - Coagulopathy
  - Uncontrolled hemorrhage
  - Increased intracranial pressure
  - Infection at the site of needle insertion
- The position of the patient is the most important part of this procedure. Make sure the patient is able to open the lumbar space for you by pushing the low of his or her back out toward you. To facilitate this, have the patient relax his or her shoulders, slouch forward toward assistant, and rest chin on chest.

VIII. Breast

33. Breast Biopsy by Fine Needle Aspiration

PURPOSE: To obtain cells for diagnosis of a benign or malignant lesion of the breast. A palpable, distinct dominant mass must be present to perform fine needle aspiration appropriately. The advantages of fine needle aspiration are:

- Easy and quick for both the patient and the doctor

- Efficient and cost-effective

- Rapid and reliable results

- Can be performed in the office

- No special equipment is required

- Easily learned technique by both physician and/or trained aspirator

- Little or no anesthesia is required

- Usually no more painful nor time consuming than a venipuncture

- Results are similar to a Pap smear

- High patient acceptance rate

- Examiner can check for cellular material immediately in the examination room

- Procedure can be repeated immediately or later

- Can aspirate multiple lesions during the same visit, placing each on a separate slide

EQUIPMENT NEEDED:

- Antiseptic skin cleanser such as povodine iodine (Betadine)

- 22-gauge disposable 1 1/2-inch needle with clear plastic hub

- 10-cc syringe of the three-finger control type or a pistol syringe holder and fitted syringe (disposable)

- 2 inch × 2 inch gauze pad for pressure after the aspiration

- Cytology slide (frosted on one end for the patient's name and/or label)

- Slide cover (optional), for use only to help smear the specimen onto the slide

- Cytology fixative

- Small self-adhesive bandage

- 1% Lidocaine without epinephrine (optional)

- 25-gauge or smaller, 5/8-inch needle

- 5-cc syringe to inject lidocaine

- Sterile gloves

TECHNIQUE:

1. Cleanse the skin around the area of the mass with antiseptic solution.

2. Put on sterile gloves.

3. Stabilize the mass between the fingers of one hand (index and middle fingers or thumb and index finger).

4. Move the mass over a rib, if possible, to further stabilize mass.

5. Compress the mass with downward pressure on the skin.

6. Inject local anesthetic, if necessary, in the form of a small skin wheal.

7. Insert the needle through the skin, using the other hand to hold the syringe with the needle attached. The needle should be sharply introduced through the skin to the level of the dominant mass.

8. Insert the needle gently into the mass (Figure 33-1).

9. Create suction (negative pressure) in the syringe.

10. Move the needle briskly back and forth within the mass at least ten times.

11. Release all of the suction in the syringe. *Very important step.*

12. Withdraw the needle gently from the mass.

13. Withdraw the needle gently from the skin.

14. Have an assistant apply firm pressure on the aspiration site with a 4 inch x 4 inch gauze for about 2 minutes.

15. Detach the needle from the syringe.

16. Fill the syringe with air.

17. Reattach the needle.

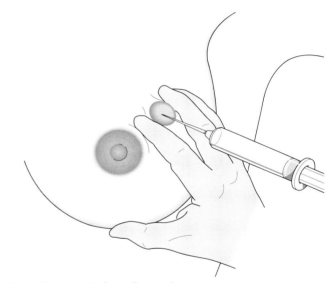

33-1 Placement of needle into breast mass.

18. Touch the needle tip at a 45° angle onto the cytology slide.

19. Eject the air in the syringe forcibly through the needle.

20. Repeat steps 15 through 19 as needed.

21. Smear the drop of tissue or fluid gently on the slide using a slide cover or the needle.

22. Look for specks of tissue on the slide and repeat the aspiration if no tissue fragments are seen.

23. Avoid air-drying, unless using the air-dry technique.

24. Label the slide with the patient's name.

25. Place the cytology fixative on the slide or place the slide in an alcohol fixative.

26. Label the slide container.

27. Send to cytology for reading.

28. Place a self-adhesive bandage over the puncture site if needed.

COMPLICATIONS:

- Complications of fine needle aspiration are infrequent and usually not serious.

- The most common complication is bleeding, which can produce gross blood in the aspirated specimen, making cellular yields very low.

- Blood at the skin surface requiring pressure for hemostasis

- Subcutaneous blood with subsequent ecchymosis or hematoma formation. If a hematoma forms there may be difficulty interpreting subsequent mammograms.

- Infection (extremely rare)

- Pneumothorax, also extremely rare when using proper technique

- Spread of tumor along needle track (theoretical)

- No epithelial cells obtained, which may cause the specimen to be inadequate for cytologic diagnosis

There are no real medical contraindications, but some may include:

- Inability to find a palpable mass or the area is only vaguely suspicious for a mass

- Presence of obvious skin infection over the mass

- Far advanced metastatic disease (relative contraindication)

- Swelling in the breast alone with no distinct mass

- Clinically vascular tumor (relative contraindication)

- Clinically benign lymph nodes (relative contraindication)

- Diagnosis previously established

Difficulties with slide preparation in the fine needle aspiration cytology of the breast include:

- Not enough cellular tissue or fluid

- Dried material on the slide (when not using air-dry technique)

- Smear too thick, making slide difficult to read

- Specimen spread too firmly, resulting in crushed cells

- Accumulation of material at slide's edge, making cells unavailable for cytologic evaluation

- Bloody material allowed to clot before smearing

Difficulties of the syringe with negative pressure technique in fine needle aspiration cytology include:

- Negative pressure suction applied after the tip of the needle is withdrawn from the mass can result in normal tissue in syringe and insufficient cells from the mass

- Needle improperly attached to the syringe

- Inadequate negative pressure can cause low yield of epithelial cells

- Too much negative pressure can aspirate gross fluid or blood into the needle or syringe, resulting in a low cytologic yield.

POST-PROCEDURE CARE:

1. Evaluate for bleeding and hematoma formation. This is the most important part of the follow up.

2. Apply pressure after the aspiration for about 2 minutes, then place a bandage.

3. Instruct the patient to contact her physician immediately if she experiences any unusual pain or evidence of infection.

4. Follow up and discuss the results of the fine needle aspiration with the patient as soon as they are available.

PEARLS/TIPS:

- Assure yourself carefully that a dominant, palpable mass is present. If there is no mass or only a vague mass, cytology yield is often minimal to negative.

- Avoid allowing gross blood into the syringe; if this occurs you may need to get a new syringe and a new needle.

- Always check for cells on the slide before fixing. If cells are scant, you may not have an adequate specimen.

- Avoid allowing the specimen to air-dry, because this may alter the results.

IX. Female Genitourinary

34. Pap Smear

34a. Conventional

PURPOSE: To examine cervical cells for precancerous changes.

EQUIPMENT NEEDED (FIGURE 34-1):

- Slide
- Fixative spray
- Speculum (plastic or metal) (Figure 34-2)
- Light source
- Device to collect sample (broom, spatula, brush)
- Large cotton-tipped (fox) swabs (optional)
- Pencil
- Lubricant (optional)
- Gloves
- Assistant (optional)

TECHNIQUE:

1. Place the patient in the supine position with legs in stirrups (dorsal lithotomy position).

2. Put on gloves.

3. Moisturize the speculum with water or a thin layer of lubricant applied up to a centimeter from the end of the speculum. Turn the speculum to an angle so that one side is at about 10 o'clock if using left hand or 2 o'clock if using right hand. This decreases the chance of urethral injury should the patient move suddenly. Advance the *closed* speculum into the vagina horizontally and downward.

4. Ensure proper lighting.

5. Open the speculum gradually with the goal of locating the cervix between the blades. Often the speculum must be repositioned and reopened several times to locate the cervix. If you cannot find the cervix, re-

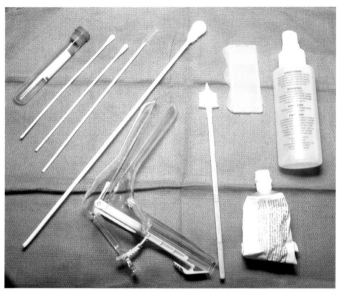

34-1 Equipment for Pap smear.

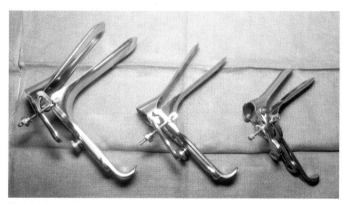

34-2 Speculums.

move the speculum, find the cervix by pelvic exam, and then reinsert the speculum.

6. Lock the speculum once the cervix is within view (in metal speculums, turn the screw clockwise; plastic speculums automatically lock).

7. Place the tip of the broom or spatula within the os of the cervix and turn it 360 degrees in a clockwise or counterclockwise direction (Figure 34-3).

8. Remove the broom or spatula and brush it back and forth on the slide (Figure 34-4). If cells from within the os are lacking, a small brush can be put directly into the os and rotated to obtain these cells. This device is also brushed onto the slide.

9. Have an assistant spray fixative onto the slide and write the patient's pertinent information on the rough end of the slide for identification.

10. Unlock and slowly remove the speculum, closing the instrument *after* the cervix is cleared.

COMPLICATIONS:

- The cervix may bleed after the specimen is obtained. Bleeding can be stopped with simple pressure.

POST-PROCEDURE CARE:

1. The patient may return to discuss Pap smear results.

PEARLS/TIPS:

- If fixative spray is not available, hair spray may be used.

- If there is a great deal of non-infectious discharge, a fox swab can be used to gently remove any discharge before the Pap smear.

- If an infectious-appearing cervicitis is apparent (cervix is erythematous or friable, or has greenish-yellow discharge), delay the Pap to another date to collect a better specimen.

- As much as possible, avoid collecting blood on the slide, because it greatly interferes with the pathologist's ability to interpret the slide.

- There are two types of speculums:

    ◆ Graves: wider and more appropriate for use in sexually active or multiparous women

    ◆ Pederson: narrower and more appropriate for women who have never had sex or who are menopausal and have atrophy of the vaginal vault

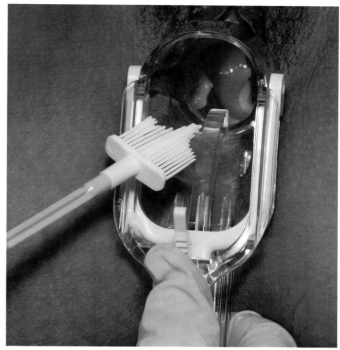

34-3 Speculum in place before obtaining sample with brush.

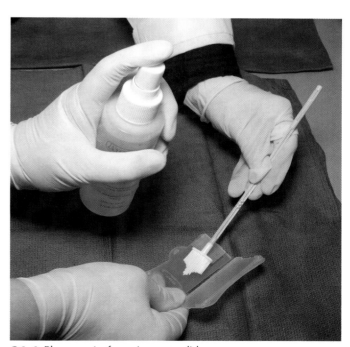

34-4 Placement of specimen on slide.

34b. Thin Prep

PURPOSE: To examine cervical cells for precancerous changes.

EQUIPMENT NEEDED:

- Speculum (plastic or metal)
- Light source
- Container with fixing solution
- Small cotton-tipped swab
- Large cotton-tipped (fox) swabs (optional)
- Lubricant (optional)
- Gloves
- Assistant (optional)

TECHNIQUE:

1. Place the patient in the supine position with legs in stirrups (dorsal lithotomy position).

2. Put on gloves.

3. Moisturize the speculum with water or a thin layer of lubricant applied up to a centimeter from the end of the speculum. Turn the speculum to an angle so that one side is at about 10 o'clock if using left hand or 2 o'clock if using right hand. This decreases the chance of urethral injury should the patient move suddenly. Advance the *closed* speculum into the vagina horizontally.

4. Ensure proper lighting.

5. Open the speculum gradually with the goal of locating the cervix between the blades. Often the speculum must be repositioned and reopened several times to locate the cervix. If you cannot find the cervix, remove the speculum, find the cervix by pelvic exam, and then reinsert the speculum.

6. Lock the speculum once the cervix is within view (in metal speculums, turn the screw clockwise; plastic speculums automatically lock).

7. Use a swab (or broom) to collect the sample from the cervix and the os, and place the specimen into a small container with fixing solution (Figure 34-5).

8. Stir the swab briskly in the sample container, then remove it. Recap the container and send it to pathology. The pathologist will then transfer the solution to a slide for microscopic examination.

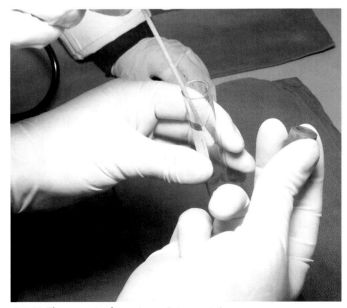

34-5 Placement of specimen into container.

9. In addition, a small cylindrical brush may be used to collect cells within the os. The brush is placed within the os and turned 360 degrees. This sample can be placed into same sample container and sent to pathology.

COMPLICATIONS:

- The cervix may bleed after the specimen is obtained. Bleeding can be stopped with simple pressure.

POST-PROCEDURE CARE:

1. The patient may return to discuss Pap smear results.

PEARLS/TIPS:

- If there is a great deal of non-infectious discharge, a fox swab can be used to gently remove any discharge before the Pap smear.

- If an infectious-appearing cervicitis is apparent, delay the Pap to another date to collect a better specimen.

- The thin-prep solution can be held for several days in the pathology lab, allowing for human papilloma virus (HPV) subtyping in the event of an abnormal Pap smear.

35. Wet Prep

PURPOSE: To examine the epithelial cells of the vagina and cervix for infectious processes.

EQUIPMENT NEEDED:

- Speculum (metal or plastic)
- Light source
- Glass slide
- Sterile saline, 1 cc in a glass test tube
- Coverslip for slide
- Cotton-tipped swab
- Microscope
- Lubricant (optional)
- Gloves

TECHNIQUE:

1. Place the patient in the supine position with legs in stirrups (dorsal lithotomy position).

2. Put on gloves.

3. Moisturize the speculum with water or a thin layer of lubricant applied up to a centimeter from the end of the speculum. Turn the speculum to an angle so that one side is at about 10 o'clock if using left hand or 2 o'clock if using right hand. This decreases the chance of urethral injury should the patient move suddenly. Advance the *closed* speculum into the vagina horizontally.

4. Ensure proper lighting.

5. Open the speculum gradually with the goal of locating the cervix between the blades. Often the speculum must be repositioned and reopened several times to locate the cervix. If you cannot find the cervix, remove the speculum, find the cervix by pelvic exam, and then reinsert the speculum.

6. Lock the speculum once the cervix is within view (in metal speculums, turn the screw clockwise; plastic ones automatically lock).

7. Use a cotton-tipped swab to obtain samples from the walls of the vagina and the cervix.

8. Place the cotton-tipped swab in the test tube containing saline or brush the swab against a prepared slide with a drop of saline on it (Figure 35-1).

9. Place a coverslip over the sample on the slide.

10. Examine the slide under a microscope for fungal hyphae and spores, trichomonads, clue cells (epithelial cells with adherent bacteria), white blood cells, and artifacts.

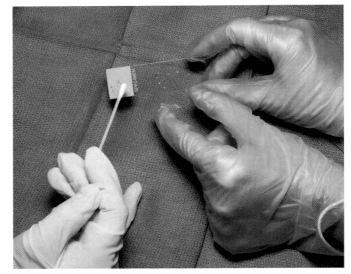

35-1 Brushing swab against slide for wet prep.

COMPLICATIONS:

- Rarely, bleeding from the vaginal walls or cervix must be stopped with pressure.

POST-PROCEDURE CARE:

1. If desired, reexamine a wet prep at a later date after treatment of any infections (yeast, bacterial).

- Make sure the sample placed on the slide is in a thin layer so that it may be easily examined under the microscope. If it is too thick, the various cells cannot be differentiated.

- Some providers place the swab in a container (test tube) of saline to be sent to a lab for examination of the cells.

36. Whiff Test

PURPOSE: To evaluate the presence of amines signifying bacterial vaginosis or trichomoniasis.

EQUIPMENT NEEDED:

- Speculum (metal or plastic)
- Light source
- Cotton-tipped swab
- Dropper with potassium hydroxide (KOH)
- Gloves

TECHNIQUE:

1. Place the patient in the supine position with legs in stirrups (dorsal lithotomy position).

2. Put on gloves.

3. Moisturize the speculum with water or a thin layer of lubricant applied up to a centimeter from the end of the speculum. Turn the speculum to an angle so that one side is at about 10 o'clock if using left hand or 2 o'clock if using right hand. This decreases the chance of urethral injury should the patient move suddenly. Advance the *closed* speculum into the vagina horizontally.

4. Ensure proper lighting.

5. Open the speculum gradually with the goal of locating the cervix between the blades. Often the speculum must be repositioned and reopened several times to locate the cervix. If you cannot find the cervix, remove the speculum, find the cervix with a pelvic exam, and then reinsert the speculum.

6. Lock the speculum once the cervix is within view (in metal speculums, turn the screw clockwise; plastic speculums automatically lock).

7. Take a swab of the vaginal walls.

8. Remove the swab and place a drop of KOH onto the swab (Figure 36-1).

9. Waft over the swab toward you with your free hand. Sniff for an odor resembling decaying fish that will be present if there is bacterial vaginosis or trichomonads present.

COMPLICATIONS:

- Rare bleeding

POST-PROCEDURE CARE:

1. Repeat the test at a later date after treatment (at provider's discretion).

PEARLS/TIPS:

- Never put the swab directly up to your nose. Use a free hand to waft the odor over to you.

- Some providers, when at the end of an exam, will remove the speculum and place the KOH directly onto the end of the speculum that contains a small amount of vaginal fluid.

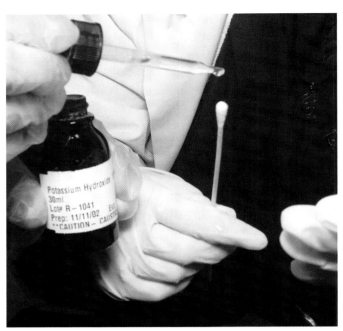

36-1 Placement of KOH onto swab.

37. KOH Slide

PURPOSE: To examine a slide that is free of epithelial cells and white blood cells (WBCs) to check for fungi.

EQUIPMENT NEEDED:

- Speculum (metal or plastic)
- Light source
- Lubricant (optional)
- Cotton-tipped swab
- Glass slide
- Coverslip
- Dropper with potassium hydroxide (KOH)
- Heat source (e.g., match or Bunsen burner)
- Gloves

TECHNIQUE:

1. Place the patient in the supine position with legs in stirrups (dorsal lithotomy position).

2. Put on gloves.

3. Moisturize the speculum with water or a thin layer of lubricant applied up to a centimeter from the end of the speculum. Turn the speculum to an angle so that one side is at about 10 o'clock if using your left hand or 2 o'clock if using your right hand. This decreases the chance of urethral injury should the patient move suddenly. Advance the *closed* speculum into the vagina horizontally.

4. Ensure proper lighting.

5. Open the speculum gradually with the goal of locating the cervix between the blades. Often the speculum must be re-positioned and re-opened several times to locate the cervix. If you cannot find the cervix, remove the speculum, find the cervix by pelvic exam, and then reinsert the speculum.

6. Lock the speculum once the cervix is within view (in metal speculums, turn the screw clockwise; plastic speculums automatically lock).

7. Use a cotton-tipped swab to collect samples from the vaginal walls.

8. Brush this swab against a slide with a drop of KOH on it.

9. Warm the slide briefly (no more than 5 seconds) with a heat source. (This step can be considered optional. Some practitioners immediately place a coverslip on the slide after Step 8.)

10. Place a coverslip on the slide once the slide has cooled sufficiently, and examine the slide under a microscope. The KOH should have broken down the cellular walls of epithelial cells and WBCs. The only identifiable parts should be fungal elements (hyphae or budding).

COMPLICATIONS:

*   Rare bleeding from the vaginal walls from taking the sample. This bleeding may be stopped with pressure.

POST-PROCEDURE CARE:

1. Repeat the test at a later date after treatment (at provider's discretion).

PEARLS/TIPS:

*   Use caution with any heat source. Make sure any safety concerns have been addressed.

38. Testing for pH

PURPOSE: To identify the pH of the vaginal fluid to aid in determining the presence of bacterial vaginosis or trichomoniasis.

EQUIPMENT NEEDED:

- Speculum (metal or plastic)
- Light source
- Lubricant (optional)
- Cotton-tipped swab
- pH paper (vaginal)
- Gloves

TECHNIQUE:

1. Place the patient in the supine position with legs in stirrups (dorsal lithotomy position).

2. Put on gloves.

3. Moisturize the speculum with water or a thin layer of lubricant applied up to a centimeter from the end of the speculum. Turn the speculum to an angle so that one side is at about 10 o'clock if using left hand or 2 o'clock if using right hand. This decreases the chance of urethral injury should the patient move suddenly. Advance the *closed* speculum into the vagina horizontally.

4. Ensure proper lighting.

5. Open the speculum gradually with the goal of locating the cervix between the blades. Often the speculum must be repositioned and reopened several times to locate the cervix. If you cannot find the cervix, remove the speculum, find the cervix by pelvic exam, then reinsert the speculum.

6. Lock the speculum once the cervix is within view (in metal speculums, turn the screw clockwise; plastic speculums automatically lock).

7. Use a cotton-tipped swab to take a sample of the vaginal walls (not the cervix).

8. Brush the swab against the pH paper.

9. Compare the color with the pH chart on the pH container to ascertain the pH (Figure 38-1). Normal vaginal pH is about 4.1 (yellow); anything over 5.0 (more orange, or toward blue) is suspicious for an infectious process. Very high—that is, basic or alkaline—pH (royal blue) often signifies trichomoniasis.

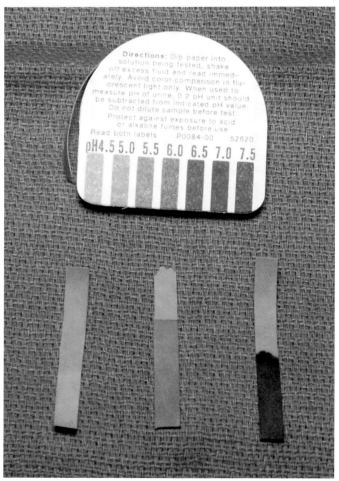

38-1 pH comparison.

COMPLICATIONS:

- Rare bleeding

POST-PROCEDURE CARE:

1. Repeat the test at a later date after treatment (at provider's discretion).

- Blood has a very alkaline pH, so avoid getting any on your swab.
- Cervical fluid is also alkaline and can interfere with the reading.

39. Collection of Gonococcal and Chlamydia Cultures

PURPOSE: To test for the presence of a *Neisseria gonorrhoeae* or *Chlamydia* infection.

EQUIPMENT NEEDED:

- Speculum (metal or plastic)
- Light source
- Gloves
- Lubricant (optional)
- Dacron swabs
- Cotton-tipped swabs
- Gonococcus (GC) plates and culture tubes
- Chlamydia culture tubes

TECHNIQUE:

1. Place the patient in the supine position with legs in stirrups (dorsal lithotomy position).

2. Put on gloves.

3. Moisturize the speculum with water or a thin layer of lubricant applied up to a centimeter from the end of the speculum. Turn the speculum to an angle so that one side is at about 10 o'clock if using left hand or 2 o'clock if using right hand. This decreases the chance of urethral injury should the patient move suddenly. Advance the *closed* speculum into the vagina horizontally.

4. Ensure proper lighting.

5. Open the speculum gradually with the goal of locating the cervix between the blades. Often the speculum must be repositioned and reopened several times to locate the cervix. If you cannot find the cervix, remove the speculum, find the cervix with a pelvic exam, and then reinsert the speculum.

6. Lock the speculum once the cervix is within view (in metal speculums, turn the screw clockwise; plastic speculums automatically lock).

7. Use a cotton-tipped swab to take a sample from the cervix and the os.

8. Brush the sample on the swab onto the GC plates and culture tubes.

9. Use an additional Dacron swab to take a sample from the cervix and the os.

10. Place the Dacron swab into the chlamydia culture tube medium.

11. Send both tests to the lab for processing. (Some media can have one swab that tests for both chlamydia and GC.)

COMPLICATIONS:

- Rare bleeding

POST-PROCEDURE CARE:

1. Culture patients for either GC or chlamydia again after treatment. A new 2002 CDC recommendation is to always "test for cures" after treating a *Chlamydia* infection.

- With many different tests, such as cultures or DNA probes, read the directions of the culture medium for the exact type of swabs to be used, and find out whether refrigeration of the sample is necessary before processing.

40. Herpes Culture

PURPOSE: To test for the presence of the herpes viruses type 1 and 2.

EQUIPMENT NEEDED:

- Light source
- Gloves
- Dacron swab
- Culture medium
- Ice

TECHNIQUE:

1. Put on gloves.

2. Place the patient in supine position with legs in stirrups (dorsal lithotomy position) to visualize the vesicles.

3. Brush any vesicles or ulcer craters with the swab.

4. Place the swab into the herpes culture container and then place it on ice (Figure 40-1).

5. Send the culture to the lab immediately. Different DNA probe tests can also have swabs taken at this time, placed in tubes, and sent to the lab.

COMPLICATIONS:

- This procedure is very painful for the patient, so get the sample as gently as possible. Often pain medication must be prescribed afterward.

POST-PROCEDURE CARE:

1. No follow up is typically indicated.

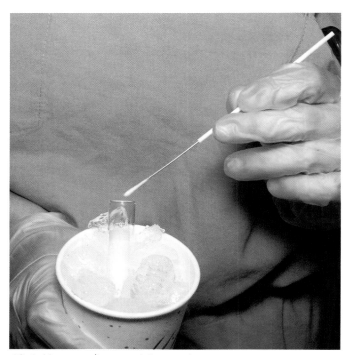

40-1 Herpes culture container on ice.

PEARLS/TIPS:

- When vesicles are present, the sensitivity of the testing is close to 90%. The sensitivity decreases when there are only ulcer craters. Once there is a scab, the sensitivity is so low that the test is not worth doing.

41. Colposcopy

PURPOSE: To examine the cervix under magnification and take biopsies of any abnormal areas that may signify human papilloma virus (HPV)-related changes or other precancerous changes.

EQUIPMENT NEEDED (FIGURE 41-1):

- Graves (large) speculum
- Colposcopy machine with light source
- Gloves
- Acetic acid
- Lugol's solution
- Monsel solution
- Large cotton-tipped (fox) swabs
- Small swabs
- Biopsy forceps
- Ring forceps
- Endocervical curettage (ECC) equipment
- Tenaculum
- 4 inch × 4 inch gauze pads
- Specimen cups with fixing solution
- Toothpicks
- Pap smear brush
- Feminine protection pads
- Exam table (adjustable bed is preferable)

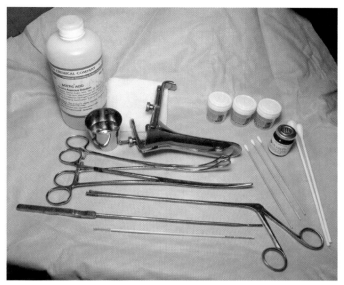

41-1 Equipment for colposcopy.

TECHNIQUE:

1. Place the patient in the supine position with legs in stirrups (dorsal lithotomy position).

2. Put on gloves.

3. Use the larger Graves speculum to find the cervix.

4. Moisturize the speculum with water or a thin layer of lubricant applied up to a centimeter from the end of the speculum. Turn the speculum to an angle so that one side is at about 10 o'clock if using left hand or 2 o'clock if using right hand. This decreases the chance of urethral injury should the patient move suddenly. Advance the *closed* speculum into the vagina horizontally.

5. Open the speculum gradually with the goal of locating the cervix between the blades. Often the speculum must be repositioned and reopened several times

to locate the cervix. If you cannot find the cervix, remove the speculum, find the cervix by pelvic exam, then reinsert the speculum.

6. Lock the speculum once the cervix is within view (in metal speculums, turn the screw clockwise; plastic speculums automatically lock). Open it wider than normal by adjusting the bottom screw. The cervix must be completely visible within the blades of the speculum.

7. Remove any mucus with fox swabs.

8. Place the colposcopy machine in front of the perineum, and focus the microscope on the cervix while looking into the eyepieces (Figure 41-2). Most machines allow different levels of magnification.

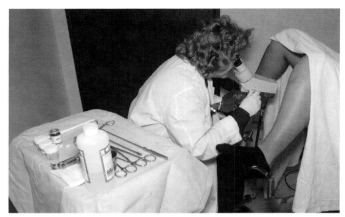

41-2 Colposcopy machine in use.

9. Place acetic acid on the cervix once the field is in view and clear of mucus. Biopsy any area around the transformation zone (the area at which the columnar cells of the cervix and the squamous cells of the vagina meet) that becomes white or has any unusual vascular patterns. Switching the light filter from normal white light to green may enhance any unusual vascular patterns.

10. Take a small pinch of the sample area using the biopsy forceps. Always warn the patient that she will feel a small pinch.

11. Place the biopsy specimen in the specimen cup by stirring the forceps gently within the cup or by tapping gently against the side of the cup. Sometimes it is necessary to use a toothpick to get the sample off the end of the forceps.

12. Repeat the process (steps 10 and 11) at any other abnormal sites.

13. Place the ECC device about 1 centimeter into the os and rotate it while pulling or pushing simultaneously. This scraping motion obtains cells from inside the os. The patient will often experience cramping. Advise the patient to place her hand over her lower abdomen and gently massage it to aid in pain control.

14. Remove the ECC, place it in a separate specimen cup, and vigorously stir it to release the cellular samples. The same brush used in Pap smears can also be inserted into the os to obtain remaining ECC samples, placed in the same cup, and kept in the cup by cutting off the top of the brush so that the lid can be replaced.

15. Stop any bleeding that may occur by using fox swabs. Monsel solution on fox or smaller swabs can be used to chemically cauterize the sites. Hold the swabs against the cervical biopsy sites for seconds to minutes to achieve hemostasis.

16. Remove the speculum after active bleeding of the area has stopped. The patient may sit up at this time.

COMPLICATIONS:

- Often there is extensive bleeding.

- Another way to achieve hemostasis is to place a 4 inch × 4 inch gauze pad in a ring forceps, and hold pressure against the cervix for several minutes.

- Monsel solution can also be added to the 4 inch × 4 inch gauze pad that is held against the cervix.

- Portable cautery is often used for hemostasis or a figure of eight stitch with 3.0 Vicryl can be placed around a bleeding site if necessary.

POST-PROCEDURE CARE:

1. Instruct the patient to follow up for a recheck of the cervix if they have any complaints of continuing bleeding or a pus-like discharge. Very rarely, cervicitis or pelvic inflammatory disease (PID) may develop, requiring antibiotic therapy.

PEARLS/TIPS:

- Lugol's solution often makes epithelial HPV changes more obvious.

- Always refer to the cervix in terms of a clock face. Therefore, the most posterior or dorsal aspect will be at 6 o'clock while the patient's right side would be at 9 o'clock.

- When taking more than one biopsy, always start with the most posterior biopsy (or lower half of the "clock" face), because a sample at 12 o'clock will cause bleeding that will obscure the field.

- Always recommend pelvic rest, meaning no sex, tampons, or douching for 2 weeks after the exam.

- Warn the patient that the mustard-colored Monsel solution, when mixed with clotted blood, resembles coffee grounds and will stain clothes permanently; pads must be worn to protect clothing. The resulting dark-brown discharge can last up to 2 weeks.

- The patient may take ibuprofen before and after the procedure to decrease cramping.

- Always check a urine or serum pregnancy test before performing a colposcopy.

- If a patient is pregnant, all but the ECC may be performed. Remember, however, that increased vascular flow will cause the bleeding to be more brisk during pregnancy. Furthermore, while obtaining consent, explain that there is a small chance of miscarriage when proceeding with the exam during pregnancy.

42. Cryotherapy

PURPOSE: To freeze the most distal layers of the cervical epithelium, eliminating any precancerous cervical changes.

EQUIPMENT NEEDED:

- *Plastic* speculum
- Gloves
- Lubricant
- Light source
- Feminine protection pads
- Cryotherapy machine with tips for cervical procedures

TECHNIQUE:

IMPORTANT NOTE: A plastic speculum is necessary in this procedure so that if the cryo tip inadvertently hits the speculum there will be no conduction of cold to any surface of the vagina.

1. Place the patient in the supine position with legs in stirrups (dorsal lithotomy position).

2. Put on gloves.

3. Moisturize the speculum with water or a thin layer of lubricant applied up to a centimeter from the end of the speculum. Turn the speculum to an angle so that one side is at about 10 o'clock if using left hand or 2 o'clock if using right hand. This decreases the chance of urethral injury should the patient move suddenly. Advance the *closed* speculum into the vagina horizontally.

4. Open the speculum gradually with the goal of locating the cervix between the blades. Often the speculum must be repositioned and reopened several times to locate the cervix. If you cannot find the cervix, remove the speculum, find the cervix by pelvic exam, then reinsert the speculum.

5. Lock the speculum once the cervix is within view. The cervix must be completely visible between the blades of the speculum.

6. Open the speculum to the fullest possible position so that the cryo tip can be easily inserted.

7. Check that the cryo gun has sufficient nitrogen.

8. Determine which size tip to place on the gun by looking at the size of the patient's cervix/cervical os. Place the cervical tip on the end of the cryo machine's gun.

9. Place the tip of the cryo gun within the speculum and then gently put the tip directly against the os (Figure 42-1).

10. Set the gun to the freeze position once the cryo tip is against the cervix.

11. Freeze the cervix for approximately 60 to 90 seconds. After this length of time, press the defrost button on the gun.

12. Allow several seconds to elapse before removing the cryo gun tip. Wait until the metal tip thaws out. This is to ensure that, if the tip of the cryo gun is still frozen to the cervix, the uterus will not be unduly pulled during removal.

13. Watch for an ice ball on the cervix after you remove the cryo tip. After 5 to 10 minutes, this ice ball will thaw and turn back to its original pink color.

14. Repeat the freezing process (steps 9 through 13). This time the cryo tip is removed along with the speculum.

15. Allow the patient to sit up if she desires.

16. Give the patient a pad to wear afterward.

COMPLICATIONS:

- Sometimes the vaginal walls are inadvertently frozen. Generally this is not a problem, but the process may need to be repeated to ensure that the cervix has been frozen for an adequate time.

- This procedure often causes substantial discomfort. The patient may massage her lower abdomen for pain control.

POST-PROCEDURE CARE:

1. Reevaluate the patient if they develop any abdominal pain, fever, and purulent discharge.

2. Arrange to see the patient after a week and remove the eschar (cellular debris) from the cervix to minimize the length of time the patient will have discharge (at the provider's discretion).

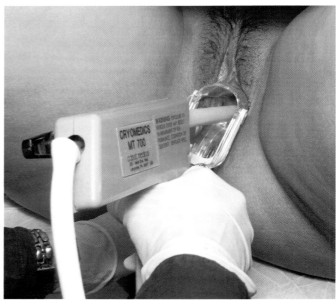

42-1 Placement of cryotherapy machine.

PEARLS/TIPS:

- Pelvic rest is necessary for 2 weeks.

- Ibuprofen may be taken before and/or after the procedure to minimize pain and cramping.

- Have the patient remain supine for several minutes after the end of the procedure to minimize any vasovagal response. A damp washcloth can be placed on the face and juice given if the patient feels faint.

- Narcotic analgesics can also be prescribed post-procedure.

43. Loop Electrosurgical Excision Procedure (LEEP)

PURPOSE: To remove the distal few millimeters of the cervix, thereby removing any precancerous tissue.

EQUIPMENT NEEDED (FIGURE 43-1):

- Speculum (metal or plastic)
- Light source
- Gloves
- Anesthetic spray (Hurricane)
- LEEP machine (Figure 43-2)
- Large cotton-tipped (fox) swabs
- Monsel solution
- Ring forceps
- 4 inch × 4 inch gauze pads
- Cautery machine
- Feminine protection pad

TECHNIQUE:

1. Place the patient in the supine position with legs in stirrups (dorsal lithotomy position).

2. Put on gloves.

3. Turn the speculum to an angle so that one side is at about 10 o'clock if using left hand or 2 o'clock if using right hand. This decreases the chance of urethral injury should the patient move suddenly. Advance the *closed* speculum into the vagina horizontally.

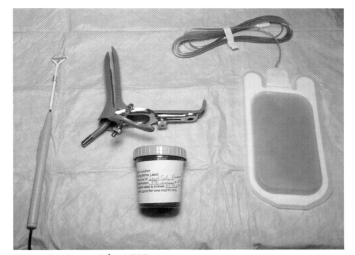

43-1 Equipment for LEEP.

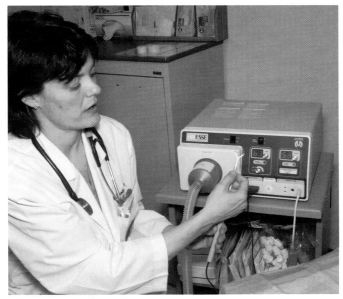

43-2 LEEP machine.

4. Open the speculum gradually with the goal of locating the cervix between the blades. Often the speculum must be repositioned and reopened several times to locate the cervix. If you cannot find the cervix, remove the speculum, find the cervix by pelvic exam, then reinsert the speculum.

5. Open the speculum and lock it once the cervix is within view (in metal speculums, turn the screw clockwise; plastic speculums automatically lock). Open it wider than normal by adjusting the bottom screw. The cervix must be easily seen between the blades of the speculum.

6. Spray the anesthetic (Hurricane) onto the cervix.

7. Bring the LEEP machine's electrical wand to the surface of the cervix and excise the distal half centimeter of the cervix. Generally about a quarter- to half-dollar sized specimen is taken. All of the area proximal to the transition zone must be taken. Because of the electrosurgical nature of the procedure, there is less bleeding than one would expect.

8. Use Monsel-containing swabs or 4 inch x 4 inch gauze pads and pressure for hemostasis. Use electrocautery also, if necessary.

9. Remove the speculum once the bleeding is stopped and ask the patient to sit up if she desires.

10. Place the cervical biopsy in a specimen cup and send it to pathology to determine whether the margins are clear of precancerous changes.

11. Give the patient a protective feminine pad for discharge.

COMPLICATIONS:

- Heavy bleeding can occur and can be stopped with cautery.

POST-PROCEDURE CARE:

1. Instruct the patient to return for removal of the eschar (at the provider's discretion).

2. Infection (cervicitis or pelvic inflammatory disease) is rare but can be treated with antibiotics.

- Pelvic rest for 2 weeks

- Ibuprofen can be taken for pain control

- Pregnancy tests must be done before the procedure

- Some providers anesthetize the cervix by injecting lidocaine instead of using a spray.

 ## 44. Urinary Catheter Insertion

PURPOSE: To obtain a sterile sample of urine for microscopic examination and culture.

EQUIPMENT NEEDED (FIGURE 44-1):

- Nonsterile gloves

- Catheter kit containing sterile gloves

- Lubrication gel with anesthetic

- Catheter connected to collection tube

- Povidone iodine (Betadine) swabs or alcohol pads

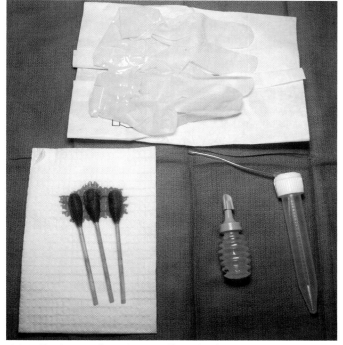

44-1 Equipment for urinary catheterization.

TECHNIQUE:

1. Put on nonsterile gloves.

2. Use Betadine, alcohol, or other cleaning swabs or pads to clean the urethral meatus.

3. Put on sterile gloves after the area is cleaned.

4. Place the sterile anesthetic lubrication gel onto the distal 3 cm of the catheter tip.

5. Open up the labial folds with your nondominant hand. This hand is now contaminated and cannot be used for anything but holding open the labia.

6. Identify the urethral opening.

7. Take the catheter with the dominant hand (usually the right) and place the tip into the urethra (Figure 44-2).

8. Advance the catheter until urine begins to flow.

9. Allow the urine to flow through the catheter into the collection tube.

10. Remove the catheter gently once the tube is nearly full, then remove the catheter from the collection tube.

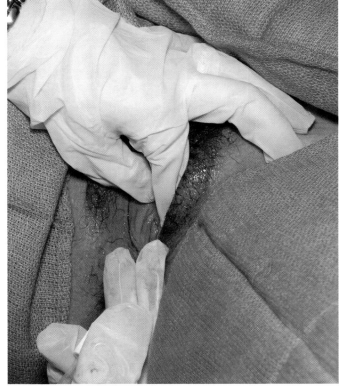

44-2 Placement of tip of catheter into urethra.

11. Close the tube and send it to the laboratory for microscopic evaluation and culture if necessary.

COMPLICATIONS:

- Often the catheter will be inadvertently placed into the vaginal introitus instead of the urethra. If this occurs, the catheter is now contaminated and must be removed. A new kit must be opened and the process begun again.

POST-PROCEDURE CARE:

1. No follow up is typically indicated.

PEARLS/TIPS:

- While still wearing the nonsterile gloves, attempt to visually differentiate the urethra from the introitus. You aren't considered sterile, so it is easier to move the labia around to look for the urethra. Once you have identified the urethra, proceed to the cleaning.

- Often the catheter has to be rotated while inserted to obtain the urine flow.

- If the patient is dehydrated, it can help to have an assistant apply suprapubic pressure to the patient to aid in the flow of urine.

45. Urinalysis

PURPOSE: To quickly ascertain if there are any elements of protein or infection in the urine specimen.

EQUIPMENT NEEDED:

- Collection container
- Cleaning pads
- Instruction sheet for patient
- Gloves
- Urine dip chemical strips

TECHNIQUE:

1. Give the patient the collection cup, cleaning pads, and instruction sheet. (The instruction sheet should tell her to separate the labia with one hand and use three cleaning swabs in order to thoroughly clean the urethra; to void the first few drops of urine into the toilet;

to stop her stream; to move the cup underneath the perineum; and to urinate the midstream flow into the container. Anywhere from a few millimeters to a full cup can be collected.) Direct her to a bathroom where she can perform the "clean catch" collection.

2. Put on gloves.

3. Place a urine dip strip within the container. All of the strip should be covered with urine.

4. Remove the dip strip and examine it. The urine dip container will have a color comparison chart on the side (Figure 45-1).

5. Compare the color of the different areas of the strip to the chart. Some must be read between 30 and 60 seconds, others at 2 minutes. The strip is placed in order of the time needed to read the colors. Glucose is first, followed by bilirubin, ketones, specific gravity, blood, pH, protein, urobilinogen, nitrites, and leukocyte esterase. A positive glucose is indicative of diabetes, and a positive ketone can indicate dehydration or diabetic ketoacidosis. Specific gravity shows the concentration of the urine. A normal pH is between 5 and 6. Anything higher than this can be evidence of infection. Protein is often seen in infections but also can indicate that the urine catch was not clean. Leukocyte esterase and nitrites indicate the presence of a urinary tract infection.

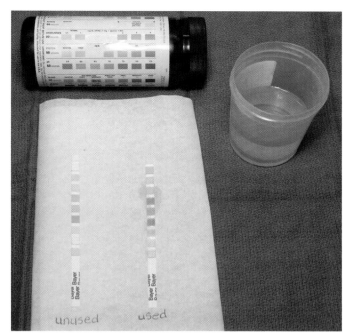

45-1 Comparison chart for urinalysis.

COMPLICATIONS:

• None

POST-PROCEDURE CARE:

1. Repeat the urine dip several days after treatment (at the provider's discretion).

PEARLS/TIPS:

• It helps to note the color, clarity, and odor of the urine.

• Urine with glucose in it can smell sweet; an infection will often look cloudy and smell bad.

• An electronic timer can help you judge when each area should be read.

• If the urine sample needs to be sent to the lab for culture or for a formal urinalysis, refrigerate it as soon as possible to maintain accuracy of results.

46. Fecal Occult Blood Test (Applies equally to men and women.)

PURPOSE: To detect blood loss from the GI tract and to screen patients who are at risk for colon cancer.

EQUIPMENT NEEDED:

- Fecal blood test card (a card impregnated with guaiac, which turns blue after oxidation by oxidants, peroxidases, or the pseudoperoxidase of hemoglobin)
- Developer
- Gloves
- Lubricant

TECHNIQUE:

1. Put on gloves.

2. Place a small amount of lubricant on the gloved index finger and perform a digital rectal exam to obtain a stool sample from the patient.

3. Smear the stool on the fecal occult blood test card where indicated.

4. Turn the card over. Place one drop of developer on the control, then one drop on each area that was smeared with the stool sample. A positive test = blue color = presence of blood.

COMPLICATIONS:

- None

POST-PROCEDURE CARE:

1. Base treatment on the results.

- Many physicians send patients home with a set of three cards to improve the sensitivity of the fecal occult blood test. The stool sample on the cards are good for only 14 days.

- Patients are usually instructed not to use nonsteroidal anti-inflammatory drugs or aspirin 7 days before obtaining a stool sample; also, 3 days before obtaining a stool sample, ask patients not to eat any red meat and not to exceed 250 mg/day of vitamin C.

- Several factors can affect the sensitivity of the fecal occult blood test:

  - Red meat can cause false positive results.

  - Vegetables that contain peroxidases can cause false positive results.

  - Iron does not affect the color on the guaiac test, but it can turn stool color dark green or black.

  - Bismuth does not affect the color on the guaiac test, but it can turn stool black.

47. Contraception

47a. Intrauterine Device (IUD) Placement

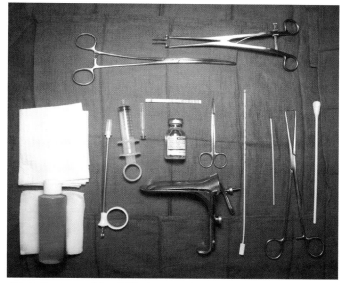

47-1 Equipment for IUD placement.

PURPOSE: The IUD provides a convenient, effective, long-term, reversible birth control method.

EQUIPMENT NEEDED (FIGURE 47-1):

- IUD, either copper or hormonal (Figure 47-2)
- Sterile speculum
- Sterile gloves
- Tenaculum
- Povidone iodine (Betadine)
- Large cotton-tipped (fox) swabs
- 1% Lidocaine without epinephrine
- Paracervical needle
- 10-mL syringe
- Uterine sound or pipelle

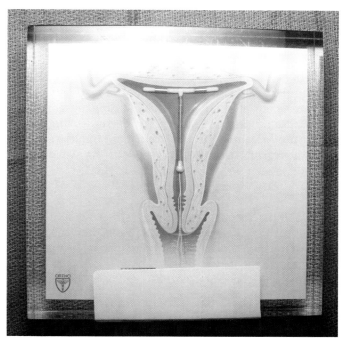

47-2 IUD.

- Sterile scissors
- Silver nitrate sticks
- Endocervical speculum
- Intrauterine forceps
- IUD hook

TECHNIQUE:

IMPORTANT NOTE: The package inserts of both the copper and the hormonal IUDs contain detailed instructions for the clinician on how to place and remove the IUD. The following procedure will discuss only placement of the copper IUD, because it is less complicated and more concise.

1. Specimens for diagnosis of infections should have been obtained *before* the procedure, and all culture results should be negative for sexually transmitted diseases. Pregnancy testing should be performed and the results returned negative.

2. Proper patient selection is important and must be based on several factors (see "Pearls/Tips" below for more detailed information).

3. Obtain informed consent, read, explained, and signed by both patient and a witness.

4. Place the patient in the supine position with legs in stirrups (dorsal lithotomy position) and perform a pelvic exam to clinically determine the size of the uterus.

5. Put on sterile gloves.

6. Moisturize the speculum with water or a thin layer of lubricant applied up to a centimeter from the end of the speculum. Turn the speculum to an angle so that one side is at about 10 o'clock if using left hand or 2 o'clock if using right hand. This decreases the chance of urethral injury should the patient move suddenly. Advance the *closed* speculum into the vagina horizontally.

7. Ensure proper lighting.

8. Open the speculum gradually with the goal of locating the cervix between the blades. Often the speculum must be repositioned and reopened several times to locate the cervix. If you cannot find the cervix, remove the speculum, find the cervix by pelvic exam, then reinsert the speculum.

9. Lock the speculum once the cervix is within view (in metal speculums, turn the screw clockwise; plastic ones automatically lock).

10. Clean the upper vagina, outer cervix, and cervical os thoroughly with an antiseptic such as povidone iodine, using a large cotton-tipped swab.

11. Anesthetize the cervix with a paracervical block using 0.5 to 1.0 mL of lidocaine without epinephrine. One may also anesthetize the tenaculum site.

12. Place the tenaculum at approximately the 12 o'clock position to stabilize the cervix and straighten the uterine axis.

13. Sound the uterus to the fundus with a uterine sound or pipelle to obtain an accurate measurement of uterine size.

14. Load the IUD into the insertion tube: Pull the IUD back through the insertion tube until the T arms are parallel to the base of the T.

15. Place the introduction tube with the IUD through the uterine cervix and into the uterus.

16. Withdraw approximately 1/4 to 1/2 cm once the introducer touches the fundus.

17. Stabilize the introducer ring at the base of the introducer, hold the ring gently against the uterine cervix, and remove the introducer tube. By doing this, the T arms will open and will be properly placed in the upper portion of the intrauterine cavity.

18. Remove the introducer completely. At this point the strings of the IUD can be seen protruding from the cervical os. Trim the strings to approximately 2 inches or 5 centimeters.

19. Remove the tenaculum. The tenaculum site may need hemostasis; if so, use the silver nitrate sticks.

20. Remove the speculum.

COMPLICATIONS:

- Uterine perforations: All perforations "start" at insertion. Clinical signs may include pain or vaginal bleeding. Perforations made by the uterine sound usually occur in the midline posterior uterine wall when there is marked flexion of the uterus. Steps to take should you suspect a perforation are: (1) remove the uterine sound; (2) watch for uterine bleeding; (3) take the patient's blood pressure and pulse; (4) assess the patient for pain; (5) check her hematocrit. If there is no bleeding, and vital signs and hematocrit are stable, the patient may be sent home with a provision for alternative contraception. If there is persistent pain or signs of other organ damage, take or refer the patient immediately to the operating room for laparoscopic evaluation. This event is extremely rare. If the IUD itself perforates the uterus, attempt to remove it by gently pulling on the strings. If you encounter resistance, stop. Send the patient to surgery for immediate laparoscopic IUD removal. If the IUD perforation is noted at a later date, arrange for elective laparoscopic removal.

- Spotting, frequent or heavy bleeding, hemorrhage, or anemia:
  - Rule out pregnancy. If the patient is pregnant, rule out ectopic pregnancy.
  - Rule out infection, especially if the patient has postcoital bleeding.
  - Rule out expulsion of IUD. Expulsion will be further detailed below.
  - Assess for anemia by checking a CBC. If the patient is anemic, check IUD placement to rule out expulsion. Provide iron supplementation in addition to addressing the cause of the anemia.
  - Offer nonsteroidal anti-inflammatory drugs (NSAIDs), to be taken during menses each month to reduce bleeding.
  - Consider replacement with hormonal IUD.

- Cramping and/or pain:
  - Rule out pregnancy, infection, or IUD expulsion.
  - Offer NSAIDs with menses or just before menses every month to reduce cramping.
  - Consider IUD removal and or use of hormonal IUD or another contraceptive method if problem persists.

- Expulsion:
  - If expulsion is confirmed (IUD can be seen by patient or clinician), rule out pregnancy.
  - If expulsion is suspected, an ultrasound or x-ray must be performed to determine IUD absence or presence and its current location. Another option is to probe the endocervical canal for the IUD using an IUD hook or intrauterine forceps. Remove if the IUD is present in the cervical canal.
  - The IUD may be replaced immediately if the patient is not pregnant.

- Strings not felt:
  - Check vagina for strings by sterile speculum exam. Access string length. If normal, reassure and reinstruct the patient on how to feel for strings.
  - If strings are missing, perform pregnancy test and perform or obtain an ultrasound to determine whether IUD has been expelled.

- Missing strings in nonpregnant patients:
  - Twist cytobrush inside cervix to snag strings, which may have become snarled in the endocervical canal.
  - Examine cervix with uterine sound, or visualize canal using an endocervical speculum.
  - Remove and offer to replace IUD if it is in the endocervix. If IUD is not in the cervical canal, attempt to remove the IUD with intrauterine forceps or IUD hook, or refer for ultrasound to localize, before attempted removal. Always provide alternative birth control. In nonpregnant patients, removal may be done under direct hysteroscopic visualization.
  - Locate the IUD with ultrasound. If it is in place, one may do nothing. If necessary, remove the IUD using ultrasound guidance.

- Missing strings in pregnant patients:
  - Rule out ectopic pregnancy; 5% to 8% of all failures with the copper IUD are ectopic pregnancies.
  - Obtain ultrasound to verify IUD in the uterus if pregnancy is intrauterine.

♦ Advise patient that she is at increased risk for preterm labor, septic abortion, and miscarriage if IUD is in the uterus. But reassure her that the fetus is not at increased risk for birth defects. One may remove the IUD at surgery if the patient desires an elective termination of pregnancy. Otherwise, plan for removal at delivery of the fetus.

♦ Reconfirm informed consent.

• Pregnancy with visible strings:

♦ Visible strings in the first trimester require you to advise the patient that removal of the IUD is indicated, to reduce the risk of spontaneous abortion and infection. However, she may decline.

♦ If the patient is having a spontaneous abortion, remove the IUD and consider antibiotic therapy for 7 days.

• Infection with IUD use:

♦ Bacterial vaginosis or candidiasis: Treat routinely.

♦ Trichomoniasis: Treat and reassess IUD candidacy.

♦ Cervicitis or PID: Give the first dose of antibiotics to achieve adequate serum levels before removing the IUD. IUD removal may not be necessary, unless there is no improvement after antibiotic therapy.

♦ Actinomycosis: Cultures of asymptomatic women with and without an IUD find that both have a three to four percent positivity rate for actinomycosis. Actinomycosis is often suggested on the Pap smear. True upper tract infection with this organism is very serious and requires at the very least prolonged intravenous antibiotic therapy with penicillin. However, fewer than half of the women with such Pap smear reports have actinomycosis, and those that do usually have asymptomatic colonization only. Examine patients for signs of PID (it can be unilateral). If the patient has no clinical evidence of upper tract involvement, three major options are available: (1) Conservative therapy, with annual Pap smears only. Advise patients to return as needed or if she develops PID symptoms. (2) Treat with antibiotic (penicillin G or tetracycline) for one month and repeat Pap smear. (3) Remove IUD and treat with antibiotic and repeat Pap smear in 1 month. Reinsert IUD if colonization has cleared and the patient so desires.

POST-PROCEDURE CARE:

1.   Give patient trimmed IUD strings, once the IUD has been placed, to learn what to check for after each menses each month. The patient is to reach into the vagina and feel for these strings to ensure that they are still in the correct place.

2.   Advise patients to return if any symptoms of pregnancy, infection or IUD loss develop. The acronym *PAINS* is used to identify early IUD warning signs.

P: Period late (pregnancy); abnormal spotting or bleeding

A: Abdominal pain or pain with intercourse

I: Infection exposure (STD); abnormal vaginal discharge

N: Not feeling well: fever, chills

S: String missing, shorter, or longer

3.   Counsel the patient on anticipated menstrual changes:

a.   The patient may take NSAIDs prophylactically for at least 2 to 3 days at the onset of the next three menses or even starting before the menses (example: ibuprofen 200–400 mg by mouth every 4 to 6 hours, starting at the beginning of the menstrual flow). She should call her clinician if bleeding becomes bothersome. General follow up for patient: Return for post IUD insertion check in about 2 1/2 months after insertion to rule out partial expulsion or other problems requiring removal (before the end of the 3 month warranty). Many clinicians prefer the patient to return for a 1-month visit and then at 2 1/2 months if any problems occur.

b.   Routine annual well woman exams for the patient. The follow-up checklist for patients using an IUD includes these questions, which should be asked on each return visit:

i.   Do you have any questions about, or problems with your IUD? Remember the acronym PAINS.

ii.   Can you feel your IUD strings; have they changed in length?

iii.   Have you or your partner had any new partners since your last visit?

iv.   Do you plan to have children, or do you plan to have more children?

- The most important part of IUD placement is the informed consent and appropriate patient selection. Be sure that the patient is a good candidate for IUD use. Patients who are monogamous and multiparous are by far the best candidates; however, nulligravid females can use an IUD with little or no problem.

- Patients with any contraindication should be strongly discouraged from IUD use. Proper patient selection is essential. Contraindications include:

  - Pregnancy

  - Known or suspected pelvic cancer

  - Undiagnosed vaginal bleeding

  - Known or suspected pelvic infection, including any sexual transmitted disease

  - Multiple sexual partners

  - Patients who are at high risk for sexually transmitted diseases

  - Certain liver disorders (copper IUD only)

  - Recent abnormal Pap smear

  - Enlarged or distorted uterine cavity such as seen with submucosal fibroids

  - Breast cancer now or in the past (hormonal IUD only)

  - Allergy to levonorgestrel, silicone, or polyethylene

- A careful and thorough pelvic examination before placing the IUD is also essential. This, along with the uterine sound and measurement of the intrauterine cavity, will prevent most of the possible complications at insertion.

- Careful, thorough counseling of the patient for possible post-insertion complications is also essential for successful IUD use.

- Consider having patient take a NSAID 1 hour before insertion. One may consider antibiotic prophylaxis, but no antibiotic treatment is required.

- Remember the acronym PAINS.

 ## 47b. IUD Removal

PURPOSE: An IUD should be removed under the following circumstances:

- Patient is actively expelling the IUD

- Infection

- Pregnancy

- IUD has expired (hormonal IUDs at 5 years; copper IUDs at 10 years)

- Complications with the IUD

- Anemia

- Patient is no longer a candidate for IUD

- Patient requests removal

EQUIPMENT NEEDED:

- Sterile gloves

- Tenaculum

- Sterile speculum

- Povidone iodine (Betadine)

- Large cotton-tipped (fox) swabs

- 1% Lidocaine without epinephrine

- Paracervical needle

- 10-cc syringe

- Silver nitrate sticks

- Endocervical speculum

- Intrauterine and/or Ring forceps

- IUD hook

TECHNIQUE:

IMPORTANT NOTE: Consider having the patient take nonsteroidal anti-inflammatory pain medication before this procedure. Prophylactic antibiotics can be used but are not strictly necessary.

1. Obtain informed consent.

2. Put on sterile gloves.

3. Moisturize the speculum with water or a thin layer of lubricant applied up to a centimeter from the end of the speculum. Turn the speculum to an angle so that one side is at about 10 o'clock if using left hand or 2 o'clock if using right hand. This decreases the chance of urethral injury should the patient move suddenly. Advance the *closed* speculum into the vagina horizontally.

4. Ensure proper lighting.

5. Open the speculum gradually with the goal of locating the cervix between the blades. Often the speculum must be readvanced and reopened several times to locate the cervix. If you cannot find the cervix, remove the speculum, find the cervix by pelvic exam, then reinsert the speculum.

6. Lock the speculum once the cervix is within view (in metal speculums, turn the screw clockwise; plastic ones automatically lock).

7. Clean the cervix, if desired, with povidone iodine.

8. Grasp the IUD strings with intrauterine forceps or a ring forceps, as close to the external os as possible.

9. Use steady but gentle traction until the IUD is removed. Some clinicians prefer to remove the IUD at the time of the menses to reduce cramping, because the cervical os is slightly opened. However, the IUD can be removed at any time during the menstrual cycle.

COMPLICATIONS:

- An IUD may become embedded, making removal difficult. Gentle rotation of the strings may free the IUD. If this technique isn't successful, intrauterine forceps or an IUD hook may be used to grasp the IUD, with or without ultrasound guidance. Hysteroscopic removal may be indicated in rare cases. If the IUD is particularly embedded, a paracervical block using 1% lidocaine reduces cramping and pain during removal.

- Broken strings. If the IUD strings are broken at the time of removal, one may use an IUD hook or intrauterine forceps to grasp and remove the IUD from the intrauterine cavity.

POST-PROCEDURE CARE:

1. Counsel patient that once an IUD is removed, baseline fertility returns rapidly. Should she not desire pregnancy immediately, an alternative form of birth control should be offered. Otherwise, she and her partner may begin attempting pregnancy as soon as they are ready.

- Consider removal of the IUD during the menses to decrease pain and cramping.

- Use very gentle and steady traction to avoid breaking the strings.

47c. Cervical Caps

PURPOSE: The cervical cap is a thimble-shaped latex device that provides a mechanical barrier to sperm migration into the cervical canal, and acts also as a chemical barrier when spermicide is applied directly to the cap.

EQUIPMENT NEEDED:

- Sterile gloves
- Vaginal speculum
- Cervical cap fitting kit
- Informed consent form

TECHNIQUE:

IMPORTANT NOTE: Patient selection is of the utmost importance. Candidates for its use include:

- Women willing and able to insert the device before coitus and to remove it later

- Women with a smooth cervix that can be fitted successfully

- Women with pelvic relaxation are usually better candidates for the cervical cap than for the diaphragm

- Women and partners who have no allergies to latex or spermicides

The cervical cap is not a good option for women who cannot be properly fitted, have a history of toxic shock syndrome, are not able to learn to insert and remove the device, have a vaginal infection or cervicitis, have known or suspected cancer of the uterus or cervix, or have a history of allergic reaction to latex or spermicides.

The cervical cap comes in four sizes with the internal diameters of 22, 25, 28, and 31 mm. The cervical cap must initially be professionally fitted by a clinician.

1. Perform a speculum examination to judge the size and contour of the cervix, to evaluate for acute cervicitis, vaginitis, and to obtain a Pap smear. (The presence of nodules, lesions, cyst, or other vaginal or cervical abnormalities preclude cap use.) Make a rough estimate of the diameter of the cervix.

2. Perform a bimanual examination to evaluate uterine size and position, and length and position of the cervix. Starting with the smallest likely cap size, squeeze the sides of the rim together and hold the cap with the dome pointing downward.

3. Apply a small amount of lubricant to the outside edge to facilitate insertion.

4. Position the patient in the dorsal lithotomy position, separate her labia, and gently insert the cap into the vagina, guide it into place until the rim slides over the sides of the cervix.

5. Check for adequate cervical coverage, proper seal, and position stability. Ensure the following:

   a. The dome of the cap completely covers the cervix.

   b. The rim of the cap tucks snugly and evenly into the vaginal fornices.

   c. No gap exists between the rim and the cervix.

   d. The cap adheres to the cervix firmly.

   e. The cap does not dislodge during the fitting exam.

6. Evaluate the fit, making a 360-degree sweep of the cap rim with the examination finger, to search for gaps or exposed parts of the cervix. If a gap is found, the rim can be pulled away with direct pressure.

7. Check the suction, after the cap has been in place for at least a minute, by pinching the excess rubber dome between the tips of two fingers and tugging. The dome should dimple but should not collapse. The cap should not be dislodged by manual manipulation, such as gently pushing and tugging on it with one or two fingers from several angles.

8. Remove the cap after a successful fitting by pushing the rim away from the cervix with one or two fingers to break the suction, and gently pull the cap out of the vagina.

9. Have the patient demonstrate her ability to insert and remove the cap.

COMPLICATIONS:

- The most common complication is an allergic reaction to latex. If this should occur, have the patient stop using the cap immediately and switch to another method.

- Spotting and/or cervical tenderness or cervical erosion can also occur with cap use. Advise the patient to stop using the cap to allow healing, and refit the patient with a larger cap after ruling out sexually transmitted diseases.

- Malodor of the device. If a patient leaves the cervical cap in for an excessive period of time it may develop a foul odor. Instruct the patient to leave the cervical cap in for shorter periods of time or replace the cap with a new one to help to alleviate the odor problem. Additionally, one may wash the cap in Listerine mouthwash and rinse thoroughly after each use.

- The most significant complication is failure to use the cap correctly, which may result in an unwanted pregnancy. The patient should be instructed to maintain the cap in place for at least 6 hours after the last ejaculation but remove it before 48 hours of continuous use.

POST-PROCEDURE CARE:

1. Instruct the patient in proper use of the cap. She should:

   a. Fill the bottom 1/3 of the enter aspect of the cap with a 2% spermicidal jelly and put the cap in before sexual intercourse.

   b. Test the fit to make sure the cervix is covered, with no gaps between the cervix and the cap. After suction develops for about a minute, check to ensure that the device does not dislodge with pressure.

   c. Keep the cap in place for at least 6 hours after last sexual intercourse.

   d. Verify correct placement of the device before repeating sexual intercourse. If multiple acts of sexual intercourse occur there is no need to add more spermicide.

2. Instruct the patient *not* to:

   a. Use the cap for more than 48 hours at a time.

   b. Use the cap if a vaginal infection is suspected.

   c. Use the cap during menses.

   d. Expose the cap to petroleum-based products such as Vaseline, baby oil, fungicidal creams, or petroleum-based antibiotic creams.

3. Instruct the patient to:

   a. Notify her clinician if the cap dislodges, as the patient may need emergency contraceptive therapy.

b. Use a backup method for the first few uses until the patient is confident of her use of the cap.

c. Combine the cervical cap and the male condom to increase pregnancy protection.

d. Remove the cap at least 2 to 3 days before Pap smears.

e. Note that after removal of the device it must be washed and rinsed with soap and water then dried and stored in a cool, dark, dry location. Rinsing in Listerine can prevent odors. Corn starch may help keep the cap dry. If Listerine or corn starch are used they must be thoroughly rinsed off before inserting the cap again.

PEARLS/TIPS:

- Be sure that the patient is properly fitted for cap use.

- Be sure that the patient is an appropriate candidate for cap use.

- Be sure that informed consent and instructions for emergency contraceptive therapy are given to the patient before beginning cap use.

- Determining proper cap size takes much trial and error before a clinician becomes confident with his or her ability to determine the size that best fits the patient.

- The FDA recommends a follow-up Pap after 3 months of cervical cap use.

47d. Diaphragm Placement

PURPOSE: The diaphragm is a rubber dome-shaped device that is filled with spermicide and placed to cover the cervix. The diaphragm provides a mechanical barrier to sperm migration into the cervical canal, and also acts as a chemical barrier when spermicide is applied directly to the diaphragm for a further method of barrier contraception.

There are three types of diaphragms available:

- Arching spring exerts pressure evenly around its rim to cover the cervix.

- Coil spring is most appropriate for women with a deep pubic arch and average vaginal tone.

- Wide seal extends inward from the rim to contain the spermicide.

EQUIPMENT NEEDED:

- Sterile gloves
- Vaginal speculum
- Diaphragm fitting kit (Figure 47-3)

TECHNIQUE:

> IMPORTANT NOTE: The technique to fit a diaphragm can be complex and takes multiple attempts to become skilled. The initial fitting must be professionally done by a clinician. Patient selection is of utmost importance. Good candidates for the use of diaphragm are:
>
> - Women who can predict when intercourse will occur.
> - Couples who are willing to interrupt sex to insert the diaphragm if it is not done before initiation of sex.
> - Highly motivated women willing to use the diaphragm with *every* sexual act.
>
> Poor candidates for the diaphragm are women who:
>
> - Have poor vaginal or perineal muscle support or certain forms of pelvic prolapse.
> - Have cervical abnormalities that prevent proper fitting.
> - Have a history of toxic shock syndrome.
> - Are not able to learn to insert and remove the device.
> - Have a history of reaction to spermicides or latex.
> - Have recurrent cystitis.
> - Have recurrent pelvic inflammatory disease.

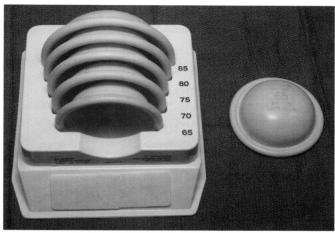

47-3 Diaphragm fitting kit.

1. Obtain informed consent.

2. Perform a speculum examination to rule out any vaginal or cervical abnormalities.

3. Perform a bimanual examination. Introduce your third finger into the posterior fornix and tilt your wrist upward until your finger contacts the symphysis pubis. Mark where your index finger contacts the symphysis. Use that measurement from the tip of the finger to where it contacted the symphysis as a measurement guide to select the size diaphragm to use.

4. Place a fitting diaphragm from the kit into the vagina.

5. Check that the diaphragm is lodged carefully behind the symphysis pubis and completely covers the cervix.

6. Have the patient bear down and visually check that the diaphragm does not move from behind the pubic arch.

7. Have the patient walk around for a few minutes in your office to test its long-term comfort.

8. Have the patient demonstrate her ability to insert and remove the diaphragm.

9. Encourage the use of a back-up method for the first few uses to insure correct use before relying exclusively on the diaphragm for protection from pregnancy.

10. Advise the patient to wear the diaphragm for 6 hours continuously before ever using it for contraception to ensure that it is comfortable and can be worn for 6 hours after intercourse.

11. Provide information on emergency contraception in advance. The patient can notify her clinician to get information.

COMPLICATIONS:

- The most common complication of the diaphragm is improper use that results in an unwanted pregnancy.

- Patients can become more prone to cystitis using a diaphragm. Instruct them to urinate postcoitally to reduce bladder colonization with vaginal bacteria.

- Allergies to latex and/or spermicide can become a problem. Discontinue use and discuss alternative methods of birth control for the patient, including a silicone diaphragm (from Mylex).

- Once a patient is fitted for her diaphragm she must learn how to check if it is placed properly and how to care for it.

- Refitting is required if the patient:

  ◆ Gains or loses 10 to 15 pounds or more

  ◆ Has pelvic surgery

  ◆ Feels pain or pressure during sexual intercourse (or if her partner does)

  ◆ Gives birth or has a spontaneous abortion

POST-PROCEDURE CARE:

1. Ask the following questions at each visit if the patient uses a diaphragm:

   a. Is the diaphragm comfortable? Do you feel excessive pressure?

   b. Do you get bladder infections often?

   c. Have you or your partner had an allergic reaction, for example burning or itching?

   d. Do you use the diaphragm consistently? If not, what keeps you from using this method every time?

   e. Do you always apply spermicide before insertion?

   f. Do you have any problems with using emergency contraception? Do you need more emergency contraception?

   g. Do you plan to have children, or do you plan to have more children?

2. Instruct the patient on the proper use of the diaphragm:

   a. Place the diaphragm before sexual intercourse. It can be placed up to 6 hours before having intercourse.

   b. Place a spermicidal cream or jelly around the rim and a small amount inside the dome of the diaphragm. The spermicide must be on the side of the diaphragm facing or in contact with the cervix. It can also be put on both sides.

   c. Insert the diaphragm by squeezing the rim of the diaphragm between their fingers and inserting it into the vagina. When the diaphragm is pushed up as far as it will go, the front part of the rim should be behind the pubic bone and should be tucked in as far up as it will comfortably go.

   d. Check that her cervix is completely covered once the diaphragm is in place. To do this she will reach inside her vagina and touch her cervix. The cervix is described to the patient as having a consistency similar to the tip of your nose. If the patient has trouble finding her cervix, she must talk to her nurse or doctor about how to place the diaphragm. Once the diaphragm is properly placed, the entire cervix will be completely covered by the rubber dome. She needs to understand that a diaphragm is not effective without a spermicide.

   e. Place a fresh supply of spermicide into the vagina if the diaphragm was inserted more than 2 hours before sex.

   f. Add more spermicide before each active intercourse, no matter how closely timed they are. To do this, the spermicide may be inserted into the vagina while the diaphragm is still in place, using the applicator that comes in the package of spermicide cream or jelly.

   g. Check that the diaphragm has not slipped out of place before and after sex.

   h. Reapply spermicide if the diaphragm is dislodged during sex.

   i. Leave the diaphragm in place for approximately 6 hours after sexual intercourse, but not more than 24 hours.

3. Teach the patient how to remove and care for the diaphragm:

   a. Remove the diaphragm by gently pulling on the front rim. It will fold and can be gently pulled out of the vagina.

   b. Wash the diaphragm using a mild soap and water. Rinse the soap off well, as soap can damage the rubber.

   c. Dry the diaphragm and place it back in its case. **Note:** The diaphragm may fade or change color over time. It can still be used unless the patient notices holes in the rubber.

   d. Check the diaphragm monthly for holes. To check for holes, hold the diaphragm up to a light and stretch the rubber gently between her fingers to look for light leaks. Another method is to fill the diaphragm with a small amount of water and check for leakage.

   e. Use only water-based lubricants and not any oil-based or petroleum jelly products; also avoid body lotions because oil can damage the rubber.

   f. Do not use talcum powder to dry the diaphragm.

4. Instruct the patient to bring her diaphragm with her each year at her annual examination. The diaphragm is generally replaced with a new one (barring any other problems with it) approximately every 2 years.

PEARLS/TIPS:

- Be sure that the patient is properly fitted for the diaphragm.

- Be sure that the patient is an appropriate candidate for diaphragm use.

- Be sure that the informed consent and instructions for emergency contraceptive therapy are given to the patient before beginning diaphragm use.

- Determining proper diaphragm size takes some trial and error until the clinician becomes confident with his or her ability to determine the size that best fits the patient.

X. Male Genitourinary

48. Reduction of Testicular Torsion

PURPOSE: To decrease the duration of ischemia and improve viability of the affected testicle.

EQUIPMENT NEEDED:

- Gloves
- Oral analgesic medication

TECHNIQUE:

IMPORTANT NOTE: Testicular torsion is usually due to a twisting of the testicle inward and toward the midline.

1. Move the testicle manually in the direction opposite the twist to relieve the pressure, i.e., twist outward and laterally.

2. Rotate the testicle 180 degrees in a clockwise direction if the testicular torsion is on the left side. If the testicular torsion is on the right side, rotate the testicle in a counterclockwise direction. This may need to be repeated in the same direction two to three times (maximum) to completely relieve the torsion. The patient should experience immediate pain relief.

3. Rotate the testicle in the opposite direction from which it was initially tried if the pain is not relieved.

COMPLICATIONS:

- Failure of procedure to provide relief

POST-PROCEDURE CARE:

1. Order an ultrasound.

2. Arrange a urology consult.

3. Consider antibiotics for treatment of epididymitis.

4. Counsel patient on bed rest for 2 to 3 days with elevation of the scrotum; athletic supporter when upright; warm tub baths.

49. Inguinal Hernia Reduction

PURPOSE: To relieve pressure and reduce risk of ischemic bowel.

EQUIPMENT NEEDED:

- Gloves
- Anesthesia (see Pearls/Tips)

TECHNIQUE:

1. Inspect the inguinal region for any masses.

2. Place a fingertip into the inguinal canal and have the patient perform a Valsalva maneuver (Figure 49-1). Have the patient do this both seated and standing. If a bulge progresses from the lateral to the medial direction against the fingertip, then this is probably an indirect inguinal hernia (Figure 49-2). If the bulge progresses from deep to superficial through the floor of the canal, then it is probably a direct inguinal hernia (Figure 49-3).

3. Administer the analgesic of choice if the mass is tender.

4. Place the patient in the supine head-lowered position (Trendelenburg) if the hernia is incarcerated, use gentle pressure on the mass directed toward the inguinal ring.

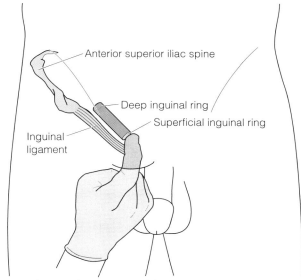

49-1 Palpation for an inguinal hernia.

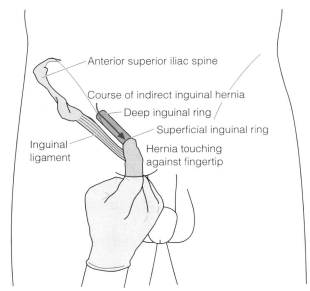

49-2 Indirect inguinal hernia.

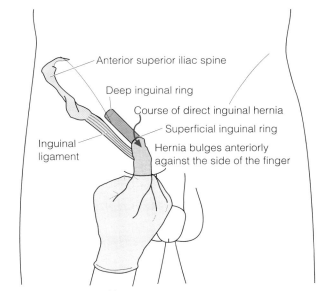

49-3 Direct inguinal hernia.

COMPLICATIONS:

- Failure to reduce hernia

POST-PROCEDURE CARE:

1. Order an ultrasound.

2. Arrange a general surgery consult.

- Administer the analgesic first. Consider using an intravenous benzodiazepine for muscle relaxation and waiting 30 to 40 minutes to see if the hernia will passively reduce.

 ## 50. Foley Catheter Insertion

PURPOSE: To measure post-void residual or urinary output on an ongoing basis (e.g., in an intensive care unit setting); or to relieve obstruction secondary to enlarged prostate, blood clots, or urethral stricture.

EQUIPMENT NEEDED (FIGURE 50-1):

- Sterile and nonsterile gloves

- Catheterization kit that includes povidone iodine (Betadine) or other cleanser; K-Y jelly or similar lubricant; Foley catheter (hollow plastic tube that comes in a variety of sizes; 16 to 18F are the most common sizes in adults, 3 to 5F in children); 5-cc syringe; sterile saline

TECHNIQUE:

1. Put on nonsterile gloves.

2. Check the patency of the bulb on the catheter by injecting 1 to 2 cc of sterile saline, then deflating it by aspirating the sterile saline back into the syringe (Figure 50-2).

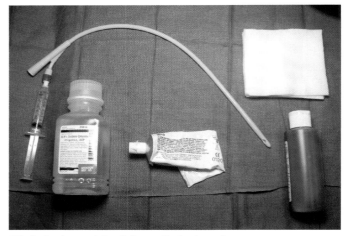

50-1 Equipment for Foley catheter insertion.

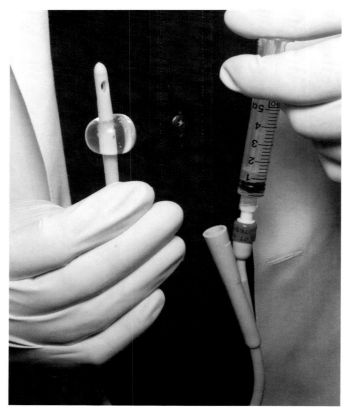

50-2 Checking patency of catheter bulb.

3. Clean the tip of the penis with cleansing agent using nonsterile gloves (Figure 50-3).

4. Put on sterile gloves.

5. Lubricate the catheter (Figure 50-4).

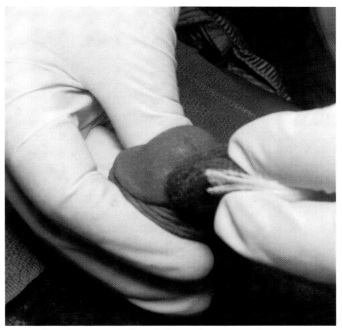

50-3 Cleaning penis before Foley catheter insertion.

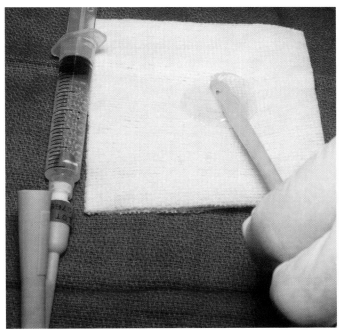

50-4 Applying lubricant to tip of Foley catheter.

6. Position the penis perpendicular to the body and pointing slightly toward the umbilicus (Figure 50-5). *Without* compressing the urethra, place the catheter in the urethral meatus, holding the catheter at the tip (Figure 50-6).

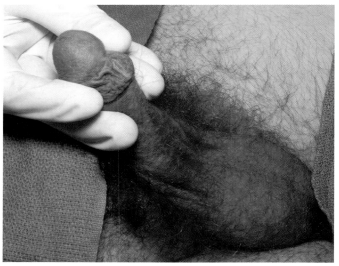

50-5 Position of penis for catheter insertion.

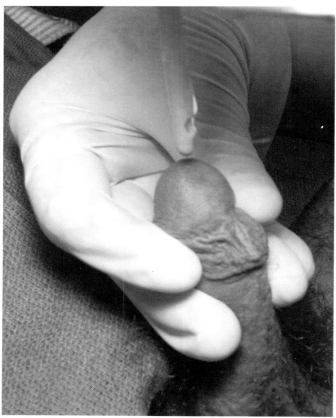

50-6 Placing catheter tip into urethral meatus.

7. Advance the catheter gently (Figure 50-7). If possible, ask the patient to take slow, deep breaths to help him relax and allow easier passage of the catheter.

8. Inject the sterile saline back into the bulb to fix the catheter into place, once the catheter is positioned and urine is draining out into the Foley bag (Figure 50-8).

COMPLICATIONS:

- Resistance to catheter insertion
- Patient discomfort
- Urinary tract infection
- Patient's manual removal of the catheter without use of the syringe

POST-PROCEDURE CARE:

1. Remove catheter as soon as possible to decrease the risk of infection.

PEARLS/TIPS:

- Apply continuous, gentle pressure if resistance occurs; if this does not relieve the resistance, then stop the procedure and consider another size or another type of catheter.

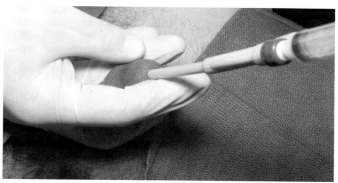

50-7 Advancement of catheter.

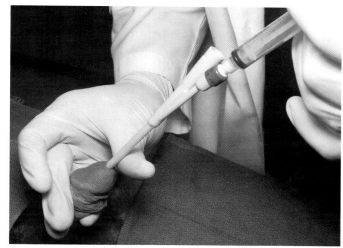

50-8 Injecting saline into catheter bulb to secure catheter in bladder.

51. Collection of Gonococcal and Chlamydia Cultures

PURPOSE: To test for the presence of a *Neisseria gonorrhoeae* or *Chlamydia* infection.

EQUIPMENT NEEDED (FIGURE 51-1):

- Sterile swab
- Culture collection medium (tubes vary among institutions)
- Gloves

TECHNIQUE:

1. Put on gloves.
2. Gently hold the penis in an upright position.
3. Insert the sterile swab into the urethral meatus. Quickly but gently rotate the swab to obtain a specimen.
4. Place the swab into the collection medium (Figure 51-2).

COMPLICATIONS:

- Patient discomfort
- Urethral trauma (rare)

POST-PROCEDURE CARE:

1. Consider immediate treatment of patient, regardless of results.
2. Counsel patient on prevention of sexually transmitted disease (STD).

PEARLS/TIPS:

- Have the patient hold his penis so that the examiner can better coordinate specimen collection.
- The yield of this collection is only good if the patient has purulent drainage from his urethra. If the patient presents for an STD workup and is asymptomatic, the chance of the test yielding a false negative result is very high.

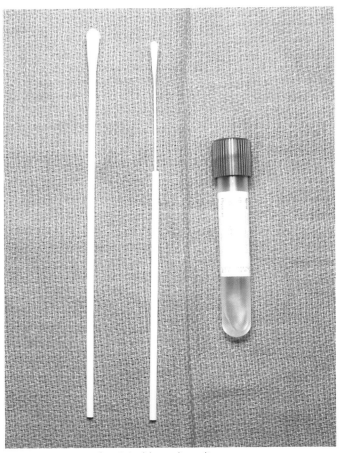

51-1 Equipment for GC-chlamydia culture.

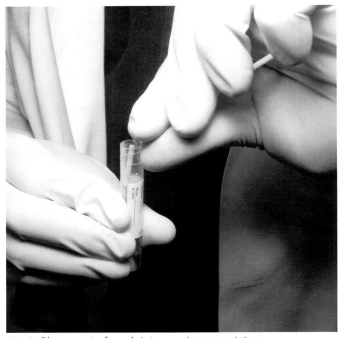

51-2 Placement of swab into specimen container.

XI. Musculoskeletal

52. Arthrocentesis

PURPOSE: Joint aspiration is indicated for pain relief and for determination of the etiology of joint complaints. For example, aspiration of a tense effusion following a traumatic knee injury can give significant relief. Joint aspirate can be evaluated to diagnose gout, infection, trauma, or other causes of joint pain. Joint injection is primarily used to deliver intra-articular corticosteroids to treat inflamed joints.

EQUIPMENT NEEDED (FIGURE 52-1):

- Sterile exam gloves
- Syringe: 3 or 5 cc for injection, 30 or 60 cc for aspiration
- Needles: 25- or 27-gauge for injection, 18- or 20-gauge for aspiration
- Topical bactericidal solution (e.g., povidone iodine)
- 1% Lidocaine without epinephrine
- 0.25% or 0.5% bupivacaine for joint injection
- Corticosteroid (injection) if needed
- Appropriate containers for lab evaluation of fluids
- Sterile dressing (4 inch x 4 inch sterile gauze)
- Hemostat

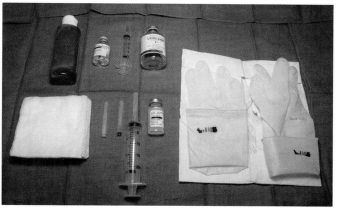

52-1 Equipment for arthrocentesis.

TECHNIQUE:

IMPORTANT NOTE: Sterile gloves should always be worn.

1. Obtain informed consent from the patient.
2. Identify the landmarks (using the guidelines below) by palpation.
3. Clean skin with bactericidal solution.
4. Don sterile gloves.

5. Anesthetize the skin and underlying tissues with 1% lidocaine without epinephrine, with a 24-gauge needle attached to 5-cc syringe.

6. Aspirate fluid using an 18- or 20-gauge needle; a smaller-gauge needle may be used for joint injection.

7. Insert the needle through the anesthetized area toward the effusion.

8. Use the hemostat to grasp the needle hub to remove and reattach the syringe if the entire syringe fills with effusion. In the same way, a syringe containing steroid solution may be attached and the same needle used.

9. Remove the needle.

10. Apply a sterile dressing after the aspiration or injection is completed.

Shoulder:

- Anterior approach: Palpate the glenohumoral joint between the coracoid process and the humoral head. Insert the needle just lateral to the coracoid process (Figure 52-2).

- Posterior approach: Identify the posterolateral aspect of the acromion (Figure 52-3). Insert the needle 2 cm distal and 2 cm medial to the posterolateral corner of the acromion and advance anteriorly and medially toward the coracoid process (Figure 52-4).

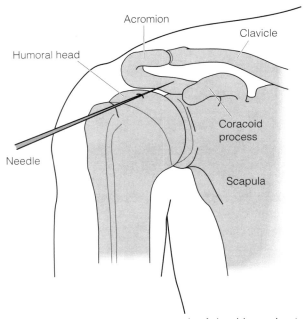

52-2 Arthrocentesis: anterior approach of shoulder and point of needle insertion.

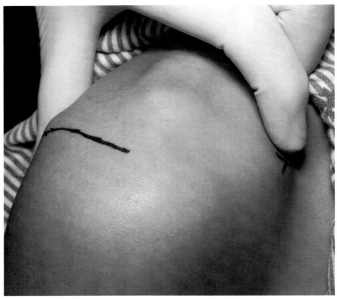

52-3 Arthrocentesis: posterior approach of shoulder.

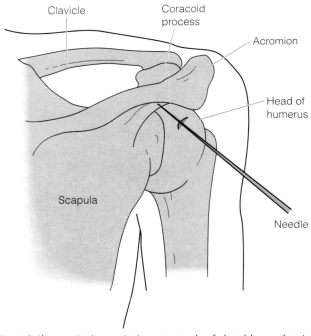

52-4 Arthrocentesis: posterior approach of shoulder and point of needle insertion.

- Subacromial space: This approach is utilized for injection of the subacromial bursa. Insert the needle 2 cm below the midpoint of the acromion and angle up 30 to 60 degrees (Figure 52-5).

Wrist:

Wrist injection is performed distal to the radius or ulna on the dorsal aspect.

- Radial aspect: The joint space can be located between the distal aspect of the radius and the medial aspect of the extensor tendon of the thumb (Figure 52-6).

- Ulnar aspect: The joint space can be located just distal to the distal ulna (Figure 52-7).

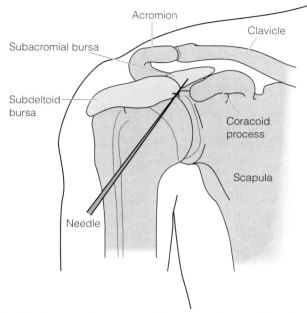

52-5 Arthrocentesis: subacromial space and point of needle insertion.

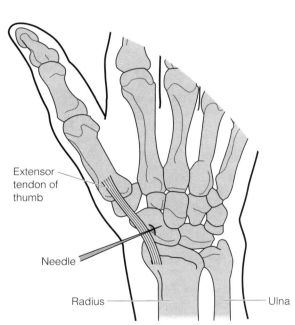

52-6 Arthrocentesis: radial aspect of the wrist and point of needle insertion.

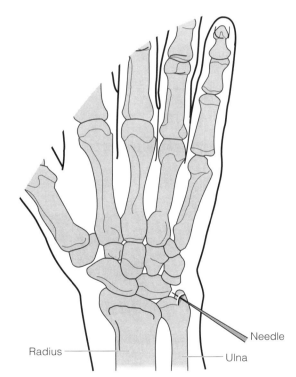

52-7 Arthrocentesis: ulnar aspect of the wrist and point of needle insertion.

Knee:

The knee is the largest and easiest joint to aspirate or inject.

- To aspirate a large effusion, use a lateral and superior approach (Figure 52-8) to avoid insertion into muscle attachments on the medial side.

- To inject the knee joint, enter the joint anteriorly over the medial joint line with the knee flexed (Figure 52-9).

Ankle:

- Place the foot at about a 45° angle of plantarflexion. Enter the ankle from the anteromedial or anterolateral direction (Figure 52-10).

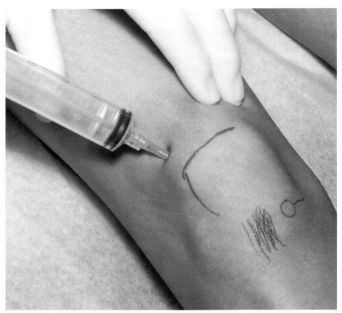

52-8 Arthrocentesis: approach for knee aspiration.

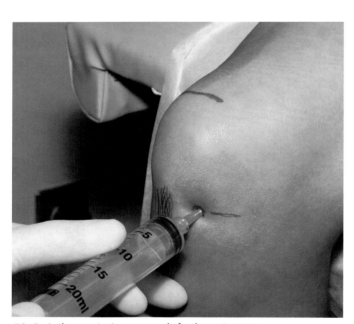

52-9 Arthrocentesis: approach for knee injection.

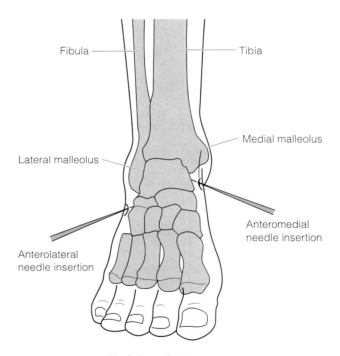

45° of plantarflexion

52-10 Arthrocentesis: ankle and anterolateral and anteromedial points of needle insertion.

Elbow:

Most elbow injections are for epicondylitis.

- Perform arthrocentesis with the patient seated, hand resting in lap. Palpate the elbow joint as a soft spot halfway between the lateral epicondyle and the tip of the olecranon (Figure 52-11).

COMPLICATIONS:

- Persistent pain, swelling, local infection, or rarely cellulitis, osteomyelitis, or systemic infection

- Steroid flare reaction can occur from steroid injection

- Local side effects including infection, subcutaneous atrophy, skin depigmentation, and tendon rupture can occur

POST-PROCEDURE CARE:

1. Base specific follow-up instructions on the diagnosis, which can often be established as soon as the joint aspirate is obtained.

2. Advise the patient that after the local anesthetic wears off, some discomfort might persist at the site of injection or aspiration that should resolve within 2 to 3 days.

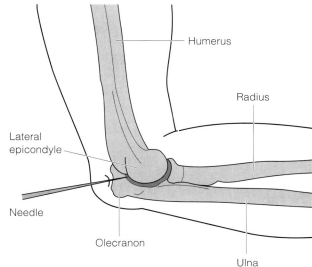

52-11 Arthrocentesis: elbow and point of needle insertion.

PEARLS/TIPS:

- Contraindications include:

    - Coagulopathy

    - Infection in the overlying skin or soft tissue

    - Allergy to medications used

    - Injection of corticosteroid into the Achilles or patellar tendons is absolutely contraindicated

53. Shoulder Reduction

PURPOSE: To relocate the shoulder to anatomic position after it is dislocated. The shoulder is the most commonly dislocated joint with trauma. If no neurologic contraindications or signs of acute fracture are seen, early reduction before the onset of muscle spasm is preferred. Anterior dislocations account for about 95% of shoulder dislocations. In the emergency department, anteroposterior (AP) and axillary radiographs will document the dislocation and rule out any fractures that could displace during the reduction maneuver.

EQUIPMENT NEEDED:

- Oxygen by nasal cannula
- Pulse oximeter if narcotics are used for anesthesia
- 100 μg fentanyl intravenously
- A bed sheet to provide countertraction
- 10- to 15-lb weight
- Assistant (for traction-countertraction)

TECHNIQUE:

1. Assess function of the axillary, musculocutaneous, median, radial, and ulnar nerves by physical exam to determine any neurological damage.

2. Apply oxygen by nasal cannula and monitor pulse oximetry if narcotics are used for anesthesia. Give fentanyl IV in a dose of 100 μg over 1 minute, then repeat every 3 to 5 minutes until adequate sedation is achieved.

3. Perform the reduction acutely on the playing field before the onset of muscle spasm if possible. Apply gentle longitudinal traction to the humerus while gradually flexing the arm forward to allow for relocation of the humeral head.

4. Perform one of the following techniques:

    a. Stimson's method: Place the patient in a prone position and extend the affected arm vertically downward from the exam table. Apply a 10- to 15-lb weight to the forearm and wrist. As the muscles relax, gently push the humeral head caudally until it reduces. It may take 15 to 20 minutes to achieve reduction (Figure 53-1).

    b. Traction-countertraction method: Place the patient in a supine position and loop a folded sheet around the patient's chest with the ends on the side opposite the injury. Have an assistant hold these ends. Next, the clinician should stand next to the patient on the same side as the injured shoulder, at or below the patient's waist. Loop a second sheet around the patient's forearm and the clinician's waist with the patient's forearm in 90 degrees of flexion. As the assistant applies countertraction, pull and gently rotate the extremity to unhinge the dislocated humeral head (Figure 53-2).

5. Reassess function of the axillary, musculocutaneous, median, radial, and ulnar nerves to determine any neurological damage.

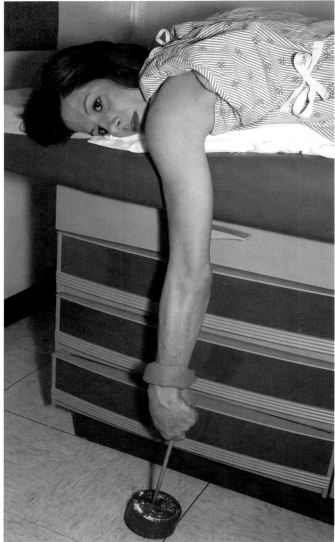

53-1 Stimson's method of shoulder reduction.

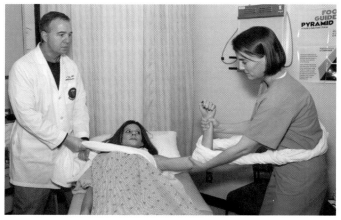

53-2 Traction-countertraction method of shoulder reduction.

COMPLICATIONS:

- Axillary nerve palsy can develop after reduction. Be sure to test motor and sensory axillary nerve function by physical examination before and after the reduction.

- It is not unusual to be unable to reduce the shoulder without general anesthesia.

- Recurrence rates with shoulder dislocations are high, especially in patients under age 30.

POST-PROCEDURE CARE:

1. Obtain postreduction AP and axillary radiographs to confirm the reduction.

2. Immobilize the arm in a sling and arrange for a follow-up appointment in 2 weeks.

3. Instruct the patient to remove his or her arm from the sling several times daily to prevent elbow stiffness.

4. Instruct the patient to start shoulder-strengthening exercises at 6 weeks. However, full range of motion should be delayed until up to 3 months in patients younger than age 30. A referral to a physical therapist can be helpful.

54. Bone Marrow Aspiration and Biopsy

PURPOSE: To evaluate bone marrow cellularity and the nature of the cells present. The evaluation of a bone marrow sample may involve morphologic examination of stained smears, cytochemistry, culture, and cell marker analysis by flow cytometry, cytogenetics, and molecular biologic studies.

EQUIPMENT NEEDED:

- Numerous types of aspiration needles are available; most are 14- to 18-gauge. The needles used for bone marrow sampling also have a stylet.

- 1% Lidocaine without epinephrine, appropriate needles (25- or 27-gauge), and syringes for local anesthetic

- Sedation, if patient apprehensive

- Antiseptic solution (e.g., povidone iodine)

- Sterile gauze pads (4 inch x 4 inch)

- Biopsy needle (for bone marrow biopsy)

- Scalpel blade, No. 11 (for biopsy)

- Sterile gloves

- Sterile syringe (for aspiration)

- Assistant

TECHNIQUE #1—ASPIRATION:

1. Sedate apprehensive patients.

2. Position patient on one side.

3. Identify the posterior superior iliac crest and make a small mark with your fingernail or surgical marking pen (Figure 54-1).

4. Clean the area with antiseptic solution.

5. Inject the anesthetic where the mark was made, making sure that the skin and periosteum are anesthetized. Allow 1 to 2 minutes for the anesthetic to produce a maximum effect.

6. Push the needle and stylet into the bone with a slight rotating motion. A "give" is felt when the marrow cavity is entered.

7. Remove the stylet from the needle and attach a sterile syringe when the marrow cavity has been entered.

8. Withdraw the plunger slowly until the first drop of marrow appears in the syringe. No more than 0.5 mL of bone marrow should be aspirated.

9. Give the sample to an assistant for preparation.

10. Reinsert the stylet, remove the needle, and apply pressure to the area when the procedure is completed.

11. Apply sterile dressing to area.

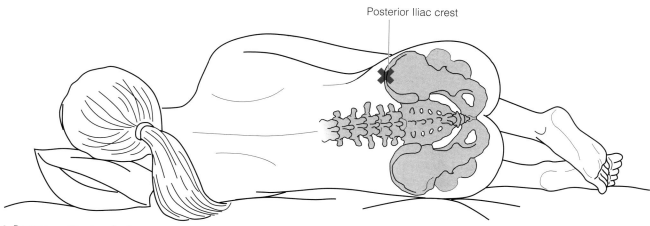

Posterior Iliac crest

54-1 Proper positioning for bone marrow aspiration and biopsy site.

TECHNIQUE #2—BIOPSY:

1. Follow steps 1 through 5 listed in "Technique #1—Aspiration," above.

2. Make an incision with a No. 11 scalpel blade.

3. Insert the biopsy needle into the bone and remove the stylet.

4. Advance the needle 1 to 2 cm.

5. Rotate the hub a few times in one direction, followed by a few times in the other direction (Figure 54-2).

6. Advance the needle minimally to break the attachment.

7. Place your thumb on the hub of the needle and extract the needle.

8. Place the bone marrow on a slide and send for appropriate tests.

9. Apply pressure to the area when the procedure is completed.

10. Apply sterile dressing to area.

COMPLICATIONS:

- Hemorrhage

- Infection

- Pulmonary emboli

POST-PROCEDURE CARE:

1. Base specific follow-up instructions on the diagnosis.

2. Instruct the patient to change dressing at least once a day, and to contact their physician if there is any indication of infection or increase in pain.

PEARLS/TIPS:

- Contraindications include:
    - Presence of hemophilia or other related disorders
    - Thrombocytopenia is *not* a contraindication

- Occasionally, bone marrow aspiration is obtained from the sternum.

- Aspiration alone is utilized to evaluate immune thrombocytopenia.

- Aspiration can also be used in a pediatric practice to evaluate chromosomal abnormalities.

- Aspiration is also indicated for follow up of leukemia.

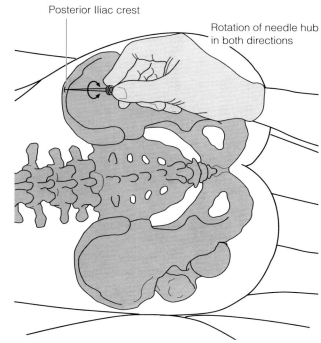

Posterior Iliac crest

Rotation of needle hub in both directions

54-2 Biopsy needle advancement in a rotating fashion.

XII. Nerves

55. Electroencephalogram (EEG)

PURPOSE: Electroencephalography (EEG) is a real-time measure of spontaneous electrical brain activity used to assess for the presence of seizure activity, encephalopathy, or life. The EEG provides information regarding the physiologic, rather than structural, characteristics of the brain. The EEG is essential for the study of patients with epilepsy and those with suspected seizure disorders. It is also useful for evaluating the cerebral effects of toxic and metabolic diseases, in studying sleep disorders, and in identifying unique disorders such as the spongiform encephalopathies.

EQUIPMENT NEEDED:

- Electrodes to detect electrical activity connected by their attached wires to the EEG system

- Collodion adhesive

- Conductive paste

- Amplifiers

- Filters to filter out artifactual rhythms

- Writer units to record the rhythms on paper, or a digital display system

TECHNIQUE:

1. Attach the small flat or cupped metal electrodes to the scalp with adhesive and conductive paste to improve contact (Figure 55-1). Most electrodes are placed using the International 10-20 System of electrode placement (each electrode is 10% or 20% away from the neighboring electrode). The EEG machine contains amplifying units capable of recording from many areas of the scalp at the same time. The electrical brain rhythms passing through cranial bones and scalp are amplified to the point where they are strong enough to move pins (paper recording), producing a waveform activity in the range of 0.5 to 30 Hz (cycles per second) (Figures 55-2 and 55-3). Paper recordings have been almost completely replaced by digital techniques that can be viewed on a computer and stored more efficiently.

2. Perform the test with the patient lying in a comfortable bed or seated in a chair for a period of 30 to 90 minutes, depending on the specific indications. During the course of the procedure, the patient can be either awake or asleep, because it is not painful.

COMPLICATIONS:

*   Although rare, activating procedures may have the ability to induce a clinical seizure.

POST-PROCEDURE CARE:

1. No follow up is typically indicated. May involve a follow-up appointment with the ordering physician.

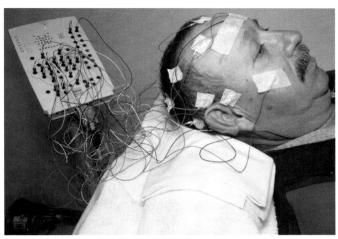

55-1 EEG equipment attached to patient.

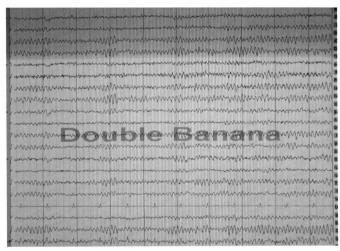

55-2 Computer EEG strip.

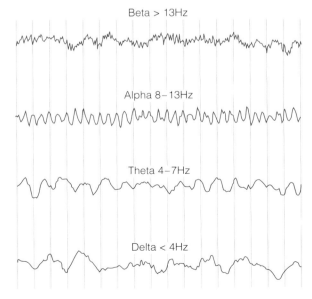

Beta > 13Hz

Alpha 8–13Hz

Theta 4–7Hz

Delta < 4Hz

Basic EEG frequencies

55-3 Basic EEG frequencies.

- Several maneuvers may increase the sensitivity of the study, such as sleep, sleep deprivation, hyperventilation, or photic stimulation with a strobe light.

- Although more difficult to perform in small children and in combative patients, there are no absolute contraindications.

56. Electromyography (EMG)

PURPOSE: Electrical activity within a discrete region of an accessible muscle can be recorded by inserting a needle electrode into it; this procedure is called electromyography (EMG), or needle examination, and it is the second of the two standard procedures utilized in the evaluation of muscle and nerve disorders. EMG is performed after nerve conduction studies (NCSs). The test is primarily used to identify abnormalities associated with disorders at different levels of the motor unit (the axon with its anterior horn cell and all connected muscle fibers).

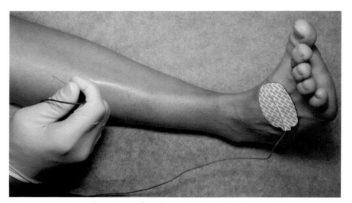

56-1 EMG: evaluation of right anterior tibialis muscle.

EQUIPMENT NEEDED:

- EMG/NCS system

- Skin cleanser (e.g., povidone cleanser)

TECHNIQUE:

1. Develop a clinical differential diagnosis and examine the results of the NCSs, then identify muscles for evaluation.

2. Cleanse the skin.

3. Perform the EMG by placing a needle electrode into selected muscles during rest or voluntary activity to record electrical activity (Figure 56-1). This activity is transmitted from the electrode through a preamplifier; it is then magnified by an amplifier to a loudspeaker for acoustic monitoring of potentials and a digital visual display for immediate display and visual monitoring. Insertional activity and spontaneous activity are measured. At each insertion site the muscle is sampled at varying depths in an "around-the-clock" fashion. Normal muscle potentials (motor unit potentials) appear as wave forms with a characteristic configuration.

COMPLICATIONS:

- Pain
- Mild bleeding and bruising at the site of insertion

POST-PROCEDURE CARE:

1. Arrange a follow-up appointment with the ordering physician.

PEARLS/TIPS:

- Normal muscle should be virtually silent. The most common form of spontaneous activity is the presence of "positive waves" and "fibrillation potentials"; these are usually seen after a muscle loses its innervation. Other forms of spontaneous activity include fasciculations and complex repetitive discharges.

- EMG evidence of denervation may not be present for up to 3 weeks after injury. In neurogenic disorders, motor units are of longer duration and of higher amplitude. Myopathic disorders are characterized by having motor units of shorter duration and smaller amplitudes.

57. Nerve Conduction Studies (NCS)

PURPOSE: Nerve conduction studies (NCSs) are the first of two standard procedures utilized in the evaluation of peripheral nerve disease; the second is electromyography (EMG). NCSs confirm the presence and extent of peripheral nerve damage. They also provide objective evidence in the evaluation of motor unit dysfunction in patients with weakness by localizing characteristic lesions of peripheral nerves and differentiating neuropathies from myopathies, identifying neuromuscular transmission defects, and evaluating motor neuron disease.

EQUIPMENT NEEDED:

- EMG/NCS system

TECHNIQUE #1—MOTOR NERVE CONDUCTION STUDIES:

IMPORTANT NOTE: Nerve conductions are performed when the physician or technician delivers an electrical stimulus over a peripheral nerve to cause depolarization of the nerve fibers and thus an action potential; the responses are displayed as wave forms on a digital visual display. NCSs are performed on motor and sensory nerves, usually in the distal portions of the limbs.

1. Place the electrical stimulator over a motor or mixed nerve.

2. Place the recording electrode over the belly of a distal muscle supplied by that nerve (Figure 57-1).

TECHNIQUE #2—SENSORY NERVE CONDUCTION STUDIES:

1. Place the electrical stimulator over a sensory nerve.

2. Place the recording electrode at a different site along the nerve. The response recorded over a muscle is known as the compound muscle action potential (CMAP) and in sensory nerves, the sensory nerve action potential (SNAP). Responses at two or more recording sites are compared; distal latencies and conduction velocities are determined. The wave form's shape, amplitude, and duration are also observed and measured (Figure 57-2).

3. Use repetitive stimulation (applying single shocks or trains of shocks at selected intervals) to confirm and differentiate defects of neuromuscular transmission.

COMPLICATIONS:

• Mild to moderate pain

POST-PROCEDURE CARE:

1. Discuss the results with the ordering physician to determine whether further studies are required.

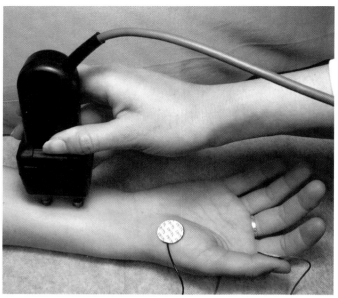

57-1 Nerve conduction study of right median nerve.

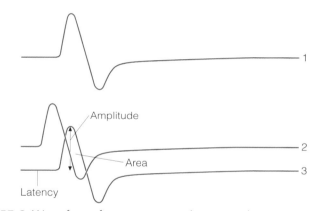

57-2 Wave forms from a nerve conduction study.

PEARLS/TIPS:

- Physiologic factors such as body temperature, age, gender, and height affect parameters.

- Low limb temperatures can lead to a false diagnosis of neuropathy.

- Demyelinating neuropathies show prolonged latencies and slowing of conduction velocities.

- Axonal neuropathies usually show normal latencies and normal or borderline normal conduction velocities.

- Localized slowing or blocks in conduction (greater than 50% reduction in amplitude) are particularly useful in the diagnosis of entrapment syndromes (e.g., of the median nerve at the wrist [carpal tunnel] or the ulnar nerve at the elbow [cubital tunnel]) and in localization of the focal lesions in vascular and inflammatory diseases of the nerves.

XIII. The Pregnant Patient

58. Fundal Height Measurement

PURPOSE: To follow the growth of the fetus during pregnancy from 16 through 38 weeks' gestation.

EQUIPMENT NEEDED:

- Measuring tape in centimeters

TECHNIQUE:

1. Place a centimeter tape measure at the pubic symphysis and measure to the top of the uterine fundus going midline over the curve of the abdomen (Figure 58-1). The number of centimeters is equal to the number of weeks of gestation, +/−3 centimeters.

COMPLICATIONS:

- None

POST-PROCEDURE CARE:

1. No follow-up care is typically indicated.

58-1 Measuring fundal height.

59. Doppler Placement for Assessing Fetal Heart Sounds

PURPOSE: To ascertain the fetal heart rate; if abnormal, it can be one of the first signs of fetal distress.

EQUIPMENT NEEDED (FIGURE 59-1):

- Doppler: An electronic device that is used to listen to fetal heart tones
- Ultrasound transmission gel or K-Y jelly

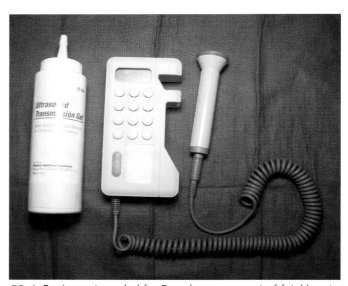

59-1 Equipment needed for Doppler assessment of fetal heart sounds (from left to right): ultrasound transmission gel and Doppler ultrasonography device.

TECHNIQUE:

> **IMPORTANT NOTE:** Normal fetal heart rate is 120 to 160 beats per minute; may be higher earlier in gestation.

1. Listen for heartbeat variability.

2. Listen for accelerations and decelerations.

3. Listen at the appropriate location (based on trimester) for fetal heart tones:

    a. First trimester: Place the doppler at or near the pubic symphysis. Tones are audible at 10 to 12 weeks' gestation.

    b. Second trimester: Search for the fetal heart tones. The easiest way is to visually split the pregnant abdomen into quadrants and use the doppler in a systematic fashion to find the fetal heart rate.

    c. Third trimester: Palpate for the fetal head, spine, and buttocks; the heartbeat should be closer to the fetal head (Figures 59-2 and 59-3).

COMPLICATIONS:

*   None

POST-PROCEDURE CARE:

1. Further evaluation of fetal condition may be necessary if fetal heart sounds are not possible to locate, or are too fast or slow.

60. Amniotic Fluid Fern (Arborization) Test

PURPOSE: The purpose of the amniotic fluid fern test is to help determine whether the amniotic sac has ruptured and amniotic fluid is leaking.

EQUIPMENT NEEDED:

*   Sterile speculum
*   Clean, dry glass slide
*   Sterile cotton-tipped swab
*   pH (nitrazine) paper
*   Microscope
*   Sterile gloves

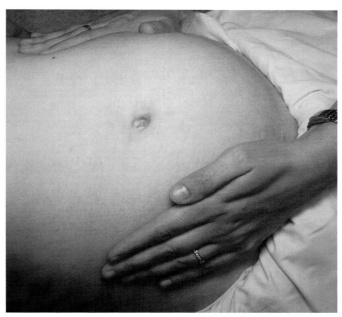

59-2 Palpating to determine fetal position.

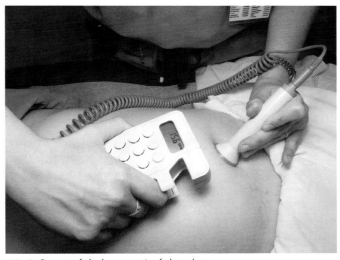

59-3 Successful placement of doppler.

TECHNIQUE:

> **IMPORTANT NOTE:** Once a patient has presented herself to the clinic or to the labor and delivery unit complaining of leaking fluid, the following procedure should be included in the determination of ruptured membranes. When amniotic fluid is placed on a clean dry slide and allowed to air dry, it produces a microscopic arborization or ferning pattern (Figure 60-1). This crystallization is due to the interaction of amniotic fluid proteins and salts, and it accurately confirms rupture of membranes in 85% to 98% of cases.

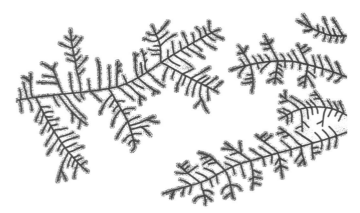

60-1 Amniotic fluid fern pattern.

1. Place the patient in the dorsal lithotomy position with her feet in the stirrups and hips and knees abducted.

2. Place the speculum in the usual fashion into the vaginal vault, gently and slowly opening it to identify the cervix.

3. Obtain a sample of fluid by soaking the sterile cotton-tipped swab in the pool from the posterior vaginal fornix.

4. Wipe the specimen onto a clean, dry glass slide.

5. Remove the speculum from the vagina.

6. Place the glass slide under a microscope under high power to search for the arborization pattern.

COMPLICATIONS:

- There are no known complications from performing an amniotic fluid fern test. The only exception may be some discomfort to the patient from the speculum placement.

POST-PROCEDURE CARE:

1. Inspect sample for arborization pattern. If arborization is noted, one can be 85% to 98% certain that the amniotic sac has been ruptured and monitoring and management of the pregnant patient should ensue, as indicated by her gestational age and condition.

- It is important to allow the fluid obtained from the vaginal vault to dry on the slide. If it is still wet, the arborization pattern will not be readily apparent.

- Avoid placing the swab into the cervical os, as cervical mucus also can produce an arborization pattern.

- Be aware that the fern test is unaffected by meconium, changes in vaginal pH, and blood-to-amniotic fluid ratios less than or equal to 1 to 10. Samples heavily contaminated with blood may not fern.

- It is helpful to have the patient cough or gently Valsalva to produce leakage of amniotic fluid from the cervical os.

- Another confirmatory test that can be done to prove rupture of the amniotic sac is the nitrazine test. Using the same cotton-tipped swab, place a drop of the amniotic fluid onto a piece of nitrazine paper. Because amniotic fluid is highly alkaline, the nitrazine paper will turn a deep blue color.

61. Internal Fetal Scalp Monitoring

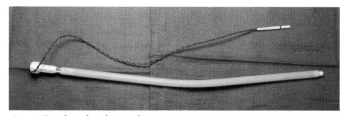

61-1 Fetal scalp electrode.

PURPOSE: To allow the clinician and/or obstetric nurse to interpret fetal monitor tracings more accurately. It is important to understand the function of the internal fetal scalp monitor. The fetal heart rate (FHR) monitor acquires, processes, and displays an electronic signal. It is also important to understand what the monitor can and cannot count. FHR tracings from a fetal scalp electrode are obtained by measuring the interval between consecutive fetal R waves (R-R interval); therefore, the fetal electrocardiogram (FECG) signal provides the clinician with a measure of the electrical activity of the fetal heart. It does not necessarily represent mechanical activity. Internal monitoring requires the spontaneous or artificial rupture of the chorioamnion (membranes), and the cervix needs to be dilated 1 to 2 centimeters, before the fetal electrode can be attached to the fetal scalp.

EQUIPMENT NEEDED:

- Fetal scalp electrode (Figure 61-1)

- Leg plate
- Fetal monitoring system to which the leg plate is connected, where the signal will be transmitted, amplified, counted, and recorded by the cardiotachometer
- Sterile gloves

TECHNIQUE:

1. Put on sterile gloves.

2. Ensure that the chorioamnion has ruptured and the cervix is dilated to 1 to 2 centimeters.

3. Identify a cartilaginous plate with your fingers inserted through the cervical os and resting against the fetal scalp. The clinician must be certain that the electrode will not be placed over the face or fetal fontanel; and if the fetus is in the breech presentation, avoid the genitalia.

4. Insert an electrode introducer next alongside the finger, to come to rest against the fetal vertex.

5. Turn the top portion of the introducer 2 1/2 to 3 times to allow the spiral electrode to become attached to the fetal scalp.

6. Remove the introducer and connect the end of the wire(s) from the electrode to the maternal leg plate that contains a ground lead and is attached to the fetal monitor. Do not attempt placement if unsure of the exact site of placement.

7. Remove the electrode by simply twisting the wires counterclockwise simultaneously; this can be done just before or after delivery of the neonate. At a cesarean section the electrode should be removed just before the delivery and not left attached or brought up through the cesarean wound.

8. Clean the area of electrode placement on the baby's scalp after delivery.

COMPLICATIONS:

- Although there is minimal potential for complications using this technique, injury to the fetal scalp is one possibility if the electrode is rotated excessively, resulting in a permanent bald spot.

- Generally, the most significant complications seen with this technique are poor placement of the electrode, failure of the electrode to establish contact, failure of the equipment to adequately transmit, amplify, and/or record the FHR tracing.

- Although placement of internal scalp electrodes allows laboring patients some additional freedom of movement, generally the patient is confined to the bed once electrodes are placed.

- A common error encountered by inexperienced clinicians is the accidental placement of the fetal scalp electrode onto the maternal cervix.

POST-PROCEDURE CARE:

IMPORTANT NOTE: Should one encounter difficulties in recording the fetal heart rate or receive information that is difficult to interpret, the first and most important immediate step is to ascertain whether the fetal scalp electrode has been placed properly onto the fetal scalp. If the fetal scalp electrode has been placed on the maternal cervix, gentle traction on the electrode will produce discomfort for the mother, and that may indicate that the electrode has been inappropriately placed.

1. Use the technique described previously and place a second electrode if it is determined that the scalp electrode needs to be removed.

2. Monitor for other potential problems such as improper connection to the leg plate, improper connection to the fetal monitor, or incorrect settings on the fetal monitor (which are usually identified by the nursing staff). A fetus with a lot of hair can cause difficult placement of the scalp electrode or erratic transmission of the FHR. Rarely, if a fetus has an excessive amount of hair, one must return to external fetal monitoring for the remainder of the labor.

3. Continue follow up once the fetal scalp electrode has been placed. This may include placement of an intrauterine pressure catheter.

- Always be sure you know the position of the fetal head to avoid placement on the face, particularly the eyes and on the fontanels; if the fetus is in the breech presentation, avoid the genitalia.

- Be sure that the membranes are completely ruptured and that the cervix is dilated at least 1 to 2 centimeters to allow passage of the fetal scalp electrode.

- Use the examination finger as a guide, and do not force the introducer of the fetal scalp electrode beyond the tip of your examination finger. Using that finger as a guide, you will be able to stabilize the introducer against the fetal scalp on top of a cartilaginous plate.

- Do not be discouraged—it often takes several attempts at placement of fetal scalp electrodes to become comfortable with this procedure.

- Consider placing an intrauterine pressure catheter before placing a fetal scalp electrode if both are to be placed, to avoid dislodging the fetal scalp electrode when the pressure catheter is placed.

- The rule of thumb is to avoid electronic fetal scalp monitoring if the patient has active herpes, active hepatitis, or active AIDS.

62. Intrauterine Pressure Catheter (IUPC) Placement

PURPOSE: To accurately measure the strength and occurrence of uterine contractions. The usual pressures observed in the pregnant uterus during active labor at term are in the range of 50 to 100 mm Hg at the peak of contractions, with a usual baseline tone of 5 to 12 mm Hg. The transducer has a pressure input and an electrical output with voltage proportional to this pressure. As the pressure in the closed chamber changes from a uterine contraction, the electrical output produces a recording of the uterine contraction on the fetal monitor strip.

EQUIPMENT NEEDED:

- Intrauterine pressure catheter, which comes prepackaged with the catheter inside the stiff plastic guide (introducer) (Figure 62-1)

- Fetal monitoring system

- Sterile gloves

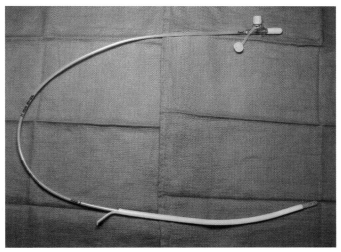

62-1 Intrauterine pressure catheter.

TECHNIQUE:

1. Put on sterile gloves.

2. Ensure that the patient is in labor with a cervix dilated at least 1 to 2 cm and a ruptured chorioamnion.

3. Place your fingers just inside the uterine cervix.

4. Move the introducer along your fingers, which you should position just inside the cervix between the fetal presenting part and the cervix.

5. Pass the introducer no farther than the tip of your fingers to prevent perforation of the uterus with the stiff plastic guide.

6. Push the intrauterine pressure catheter gently up through the guide and into the uterine cavity until it is about halfway up, a distance of around 18 inches from the tip of the catheter to the labia majora. Currently, most commercial manufactures place a marker at about the 18-inch level, using the word STOP in capital letters. The STOP should be advanced no further than the labia majora.

7. Attach the placed catheter to the electrode, which is then plugged into the fetal monitor.

COMPLICATIONS:

- Uncommonly, cord prolapse, endometritis, uterine rupture (when introducing the catheter), or disruption of placental implantation (abruption)

- If the tracing does not show symmetrical smooth pressure changes in association with the patient's contractions, the catheter may be plugged or kinked.

- If a kink or a plug (with a blood clot or a piece of the amnion) is suspected, the catheter can be flushed with normal saline.

- If flushing the catheter does not produce the proper contraction pattern, consider pulling the catheter out 2 to 3 cm to relieve any kinking.

- Occasionally, it is necessary to replace the catheter if a good recording does not result from these simple manipulations.

POST-PROCEDURE CARE:

1. Ensure that the catheter is working by flushing it to relieve kinking or dislodge plugs when necessary. Troubleshooting is the most important part of follow-up care.

2. Consider the possibility of a placental abruption and address this issue immediately if the fetus has a sudden deceleration, the patient has excessive bleeding, or you see evidence of continuous contractions or hyperstimulation.

3. Consider a uterine rupture if there is a sudden loss in the intrauterine pressure accompanied by excessive pain and/or bleeding.

4. Use the intrauterine pressure catheter to assist in evaluating adequacy of the labor pattern and make diagnostic management decisions based on the intrauterine pressure and contraction pattern.

PEARLS/TIPS:

- Before placing the intrauterine pressure catheter, be sure that the cervix is dilated at least 1 to 2 cm.

- Avoid placing the stiff plastic guide more than 1 cm inside the cervix or beyond the examination finger.

- The advancement of the pressure catheter should be fairly easy with minimal resistance. Should one find excessive resistance, stop the introduction and reposition to avoid injury to the fetus or the uterus.

- Consider placing IUPC *before* placing electronic fetal scalp leads to avoid displacing the fetal scalp leads during placement of the IUPC.

XIV. Infants and Children

63. Giving Injections

63a. Intramuscular (IM) Injection

PURPOSE: To administer medication or vaccine for absorption by the vasculature of the muscle.

EQUIPMENT NEEDED:

- For infants and children less than 100 pounds: 1-inch needle

- For children and adolescents more than 100 pounds: 1 1/4- to 1 1/2-inch needle

- Needle diameter: 22- to 25-gauge (Smaller diameter needles, such as 25- to 30-gauge, cause less discomfort but are not suitable for viscous medications, and bend easily.)

- Syringes, 3-cc

- Alcohol pads

- Disposable gloves

- Sterile gauze dressing and tape or self-adhesive bandage

TECHNIQUE—LOCATING THE INJECTION SITE:

IMPORTANT NOTE: The volume of medication must be considered before planning an IM injection. No more than 1 mL should be injected intramuscularly in infants and small children. Older children and small adults should receive no more than 2 mL intramuscularly. Well-developed, normal-sized adults can safely tolerate up to 3 mL in large muscles such as the vastus lateralis or dorsogluteal muscles. Selection of an IM injection site should be based on the volume and character of the medication to be injected, the integrity of the selected muscle, and number of injections to be given during a therapeutic course. Generally, the larger the volume of medication, the larger the selected muscle should be.

There are four preferred IM injection sites, each with unique advantages and disadvantages:

Vastus lateralis muscle (VL):

The VL is typically a large muscle on the anterior lateral aspect of the thigh and is the preferred IM injection site for infants. It is relatively free of large blood vessels and nerves and is easily accessible in young children.

1. Identify the VL by palpating the greater trochanter of the femur and the knee joint and dividing the distance into the three quadrants.

2. Administer the IM injection in the middle third quadrant. When injecting into the VL, the needle should be perpendicular to the thigh in young children. In infants, the needle should be inserted at a 45° angle toward the knee (Figure 63-1).

Ventrogluteal muscle (VG):

The VG muscle injection site is a deep muscular site that can be easily localized with prominent, bony landmarks. VG injections are generally less painful than VL injections.

1. Identify the VG injection site by placing your palm over the patient's greater trochanter, with the index finger over the anterior superior iliac spine and the adjacent middle finger over the posterior iliac crest, forming a V shape with the spread fingers.

2. Insert the needle into the center of the V, perpendicular to the site but with a slight angle toward the iliac crest. Slight flexion of the knee and hip can help to relax the muscle (Figure 63-2).

Dorsogluteal muscle (DG):

The DG has traditionally been a favorite for injections, but caution must be maintained because of the presence of the sciatic nerve and large blood vessels in this region. The DG site should not be used in children less than 3 years of age. The DG injection site is located in the outer region of the upper outer quadrant of the buttock, 6 to 8 cm below the posterior iliac crest.

1. Approximate the DG injection site by drawing a line between the greater trochanter and posterior superior iliac spine. The injection site should be superior and lateral to this line, into the gluteus maximus or medius muscle.

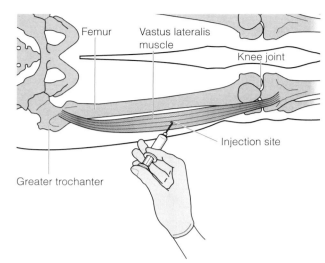

63-1 Intramuscular injection: vastus lateralis muscle and injection site.

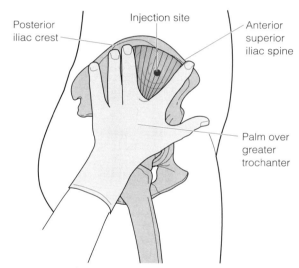

63-2 Intramuscular injection: ventrogluteal muscle and injection site.

2. Insert the needle perpendicular to the skin (Figure 63-3).

Deltoid muscle (DM):

The DM is poorly developed in young children, and is primarily used for vaccinations in adolescents and adults. Only small volumes (0.5–1.0 mL) should be injected into this site. Intramuscular injections into the DM should only be in the upper third of the muscle to avoid the brachial artery and radial nerve.

1. Arrange the patient's arm so it is relaxed and flexed at the elbow.

2. Palpate the acromion process; the injection site should be 2 to 3 finger breadths (3 to 4 cm) below the lower border of the acromion.

3. Insert the needle perpendicular to the site, angled slightly toward the shoulder (Figure 63-4).

TECHNIQUE—DELIVERING THE INJECTION:

1. Clean the skin of the selected injection site with alcohol and allow it to dry before any intramuscular injection.

2. Grasp the chosen muscle firmly while spreading the skin between the thumb and index finger to displace subcutaneous tissue.

3. Insert the needle quickly and aspirate for blood (Figure 63-5). If blood is aspirated, the needle should be removed and changed before reinsertion.

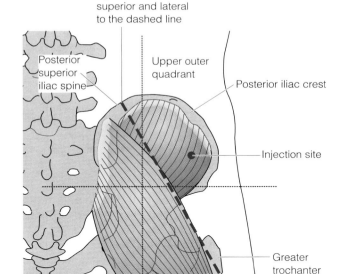

63-3 Intramuscular injection: dorsogluteal muscle and injection site.

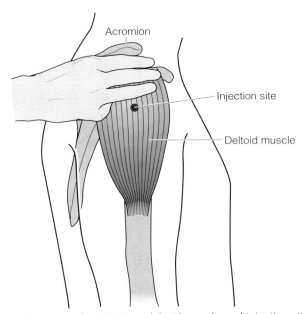

63-4 Intramuscular injection: deltoid muscle and injection site.

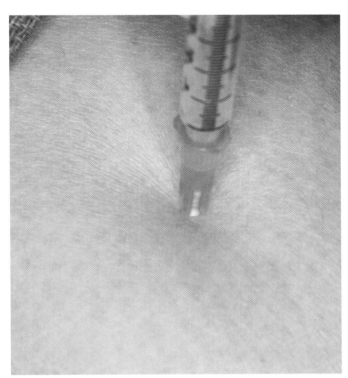

63-5 Insertion of needle for IM injection.

4. Inject the medication slowly over 15 to 20 seconds if no blood is aspirated.

5. Remove the needle quickly, then apply firm pressure with a sterile gauze. A small dressing may be applied to prevent bleeding.

COMPLICATIONS:

- Thrombosis of blood vessels or nerve damage from inadvertent administration of medication into a blood vessel or nerve

- Osteomyelitis

- Hematoma or bleeding

- Pain or discomfort at the injection site

- Subcutaneous infection of the injection site

- Adverse reactions from the medication or vaccine administered

POST-PROCEDURE CARE:

1. Base follow up individually on the medication or vaccination administered intramuscularly.

2. Instruct the patient (or parent or guardian) to return promptly if any persistent marked erythema or worsening discomfort develops at the intramuscular injection site.

PEARLS/TIPS:

- Always verify that the medication or vaccination to be administered can be given intramuscularly. Many drugs, such as vancomycin, have an oral form and an intravenous form, but cannot be given intramuscularly.

- If possible, IM medications should be warmed to room temperature before administration to minimize discomfort.

- Viscous IM medications such as benzathine penicillin are so thick that it is not possible to identify inadvertent insertion into a blood vessel by aspiration. Care should be given to administer these medications well away from large blood vessels.

- After cleansing the skin with an alcohol solution, briefly allow the alcohol to dry before giving the injection. Failing to permit the alcohol to dry can cause additional discomfort.

63b. Subcutaneous (SQ) Injection

PURPOSE: To administer medications or vaccines into vascular connective tissue below the dermis.

EQUIPMENT NEEDED:

- Syringe, 1- to 2-cc
- Needle, 25- to 27-gauge
- Needle of 3/8 to 5/8 inch in length (A useful guide is to estimate needle length as half the width of the skin fold.)
- Alcohol swab
- Disposable gloves
- Self-adhesive bandage

TECHNIQUE:

IMPORTANT NOTE: Only water-soluble medications in small volumes (less than 0.5 mL) should be administered by SQ injection. The ideal SQ injection site depends on the medication, patient nutrition, and frequency of injections. Preferred SQ injection sites include the outer aspect of the upper arms, the anterior aspect of the upper thighs, and abdomen between the inferior costal margin and superior iliac crest. The abdomen is the preferred site for SQ injections for heparin, and in thin patients with little subcutaneous tissue. If SQ injections are to be given routinely, as in SQ administration of insulin in diabetes mellitus, injection sites should be rotated to prevent tissue atrophy (lipodystrophy), which can adversely affect absorption of the medication.

1. Inspect the injection site; it should be free from infection and scar tissue.

2. Clean the site with an alcohol swab and briefly allow to dry.

3. Grasp the skin of the injection site with the nondominant hand.

4. Insert the needle with the bevel up at a 45° angle (Figure 63-6). In obese patients, insert the needle at a 90° angle.

5. Aspirate for blood with the syringe. If blood is aspirated, the needle should be removed and discarded with the medication.

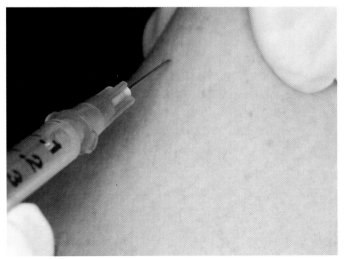

63-6 Position of needle for subcutaneous injection.

6. If blood is not aspirated inject the medication slowly.

7. Withdraw the needle and dispose of it.

8. Apply a small adhesive bandage to prevent bleeding.

COMPLICATIONS:

- Hematoma or bleeding

- Pain or discomfort at the injection site

- Subcutaneous infection at the injection site

- Thrombosis of blood vessels or nerve damage from inadvertent administration of medication into a blood vessel or nerve

- Adverse reactions from the medication or vaccine administered

- With frequent SQ injections in the same region, hypertrophy of the skin and lipodystrophy can develop.

POST-PROCEDURE CARE:

1. Base follow up individually upon the medication or vaccine administered subcutaneously.

2. Instruct the patients (or parent or guardian) to return promptly if any marked erythema, edema, or significant pain develops at the subcutaneous injection site.

PEARLS/TIPS:

- Frequent administration of SQ injections of low-dose heparin has a high association with bruising independent of injection technique.

- Rotation of injection sites for SQ insulin injections to prevent lipodystrophy should be heavily emphasized as part of a diabetes education program.

- Place the self-adhesive bandage at the base of your syringe so that it is readily available to place on the skin immediately after withdrawal of the needle.

64. Rectal Temperature

PURPOSE: Measurement of body temperature. Currently a wide array of electronic thermometers is available in addition to the traditional mercury in a glass thermometer. Electronic thermometers have become the preferred device for measuring rectal temperature, because the disposable plastic sheath is much less likely to break and damage the rectal mucosa.

EQUIPMENT NEEDED:

- Thermometer (mercury in glass, or electronic) (Figure 64-1)

- Lubricant gel (for mercury in glass thermometers only)

- Disposable gloves

TECHNIQUE #1—MERCURY IN GLASS THERMOMETERS:

IMPORTANT NOTE: Before starting the procedure, the mercury should read less than 96°F (35.5°C). If mercury is above this level, rapidly shake the thermometer downward until the mercury is below 96°F.

1. Place a small amount of lubricant over the blunt bulb of the thermometer.

2. Position the patient with the legs flexed, preferably on his or her side.

3. Spread the buttocks to expose the anus.

4. Insert the bulb of the thermometer 1.5 to 2.0 cm into the infant or child patient's anus, and 3.0 to 3.5 cm in an adult (Figure 64-2). Never "force" it if resistance is met.

5. Wait for temperature reading. There is no consensus on the optimal duration of time for mercury in a glass thermometer to remain in place. Most authorities agree that an insertion time of 2 minutes is generally adequate for a reliable measurement.

6. Remove the thermometer after a minimum of 2 minutes and read the temperature measurement at eye level.

7. Wipe the anal area clean of lubricant or stool.

8. Wipe the thermometer clean and place it in a sterilizing solution.

64-1 Rectal thermometer.

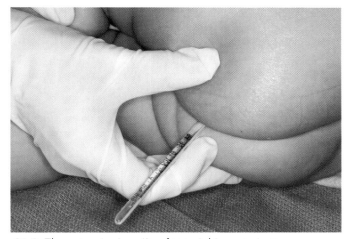

64-2 Thermometer insertion for rectal temperature.

TECHNIQUE #2—ELECTRONIC THERMOMETERS:

IMPORTANT NOTE: An electronic temperature-measuring device utilizes a temperature-sensitive probe covered by a disposable plastic sheath.

1. Place the sheath over the probe and apply lubricant gel.

2. Position the patient with the legs flexed, preferably on their side, and insert the probe tip into the anus 1.5 to 2.0 cm in an infant and 3.0 to 3.5 cm in an adult. Never "force" it if resistance is met.

3. Wait for temperature reading. The duration of time for a measurement varies among devices, but is generally much more rapid than with a glass thermometer. A digital measurement will be displayed on the unit.

4. Remove the probe and discard the plastic sheath into a hazardous waste container.

5. Wipe the anal area clean of any stool or lubricant gel.

COMPLICATIONS:

- The greatest potential hazard is breakage of a glass thermometer with laceration to rectal tissue, musculature, and nerves.

- Risk of rectal perforation

- If a mercury glass thermometer is advanced too far in the rectum, it may not be manually retrievable, and will require endoscopic removal.

- Perirectal abscess, translocation of gut bacteria into the blood stream in neutropenic patients

POST-PROCEDURE CARE:

1. No follow up is typically indicated. Any rectal discomfort, bleeding, or erythema should be promptly evaluated.

PEARLS/TIPS:

- Rectal temperature measurement should *never* be performed in persons who are neutropenic (absolute neutrophil count of less than 1500) due to risk of translocation of gastrointestinal bacteria into the blood stream.

- If resistance is met while placing the thermometer, do *not* attempt to force the thermometer past the resistance.

- When performing a rectal temperature reading in infants, it is advisable to place a drape over the genitalia, because placement of the thermometer often stimulates urination.

- Rectal temperature measurements should not be performed in patients who have had prior rectal surgery.

65. Throat Swab

PURPOSE: To obtain cultures from the oropharynx or a sample for a rapid detection assay for group A streptococci.

EQUIPMENT NEEDED:

- Appropriate culturette or swab: Rayon-tipped cotton swabs or Dacron swabs are most commonly used for cultures of group A streptococci. Viral pharyngeal cultures should also be collected with a Dacron swab. Calcium alginate swabs are most useful for cultures of chlamydiae.

- Multiple kits are available for rapid streptococcal antigen-detection containing specific swabs for use with the individual kit.

- Tongue blade (optional)

- Light source

TECHNIQUE:

IMPORTANT NOTE: Rapid streptococcal antigen-detection tests have lower sensitivity than specificity. Therefore, when performing one of these tests it is advisable to obtain a concomitant throat culture swab for group A streptococci also. If the rapid streptococcal antigen test is positive, the throat culture swab for group A streptococci can be discarded. If the rapid streptococcal antigen test is negative or indeterminate, the throat culture swab should be sent for confirmation.

1. Position the patient upright and leaning forward, to slightly lessen the gag reflex that can be caused by obtaining the throat swab.

2. Ensure proper visualization of the posterior pharynx and tonsils with an adequate light source. This is essential to obtaining an appropriate sample (Figure 65-1).

3. Determine the appropriate culturette or swab before performing the procedure.

4. Have the patient open his or her mouth with the tongue extended (Figure 65-2).

5. Apply the swab firmly to both tonsillar surfaces and the posterior pharyngeal wall, avoiding contact with the tongue or saliva.

6. Swab the tonsillar pillars, if the tonsils have been removed or atrophied.

7. Have the parent or assistant gently restrain combative children, and use a tongue blade to depress the tongue to obtain the sample.

COMPLICATIONS:

- Gagging or emesis

POST-PROCEDURE CARE:

1. No follow up is typically indicated.

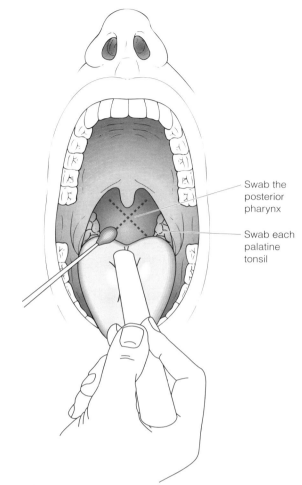

Swab the posterior pharynx

Swab each palatine tonsil

65-1 Throat swab locations.

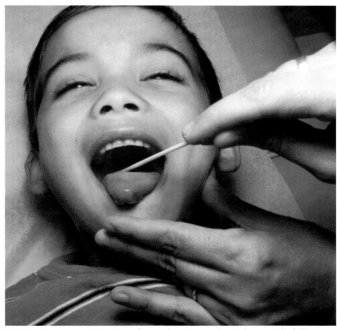

65-2 Proper positioning for a throat swab with mouth fully open and tongue extended.

PEARLS/TIPS:

- To obtain a concomitant rapid antigen-detection swab and throat culture swab, the two swabs can be placed adjacently when the procedure is performed.

- In patients with an active gag reflex, have an emesis basin handy.

- Throat cultures and even use of a tongue blade for examination of the retropharynx are contraindicated if epiglottitis is suspected.

66. Heel Stick

PURPOSE: To obtain a small peripheral venous blood sample in infants.

EQUIPMENT NEEDED (FIGURE 66-1):

- Warm compresses or infant heel warmer packet
- Alcohol pads
- Automatic lancet device
- Sterile gauze dressing

TECHNIQUE:

IMPORTANT NOTE: The puncture site should be on either lateral aspect of the heel (Figure 66-2). The medial aspect of the heel should be avoided to minimize the risk of penetration into the calcaneous bone. The depth of the puncture should be less than 2.5 mm.

1. Apply a warm compress or infant heel warmer to the heel for approximately 5 minutes to induce vasodilation and increase blood flow before taking a blood sample.

2. Clean the lower heel with an alcohol solution and allow it to dry.

3. Use an automatic lancet device to puncture the skin. Automated devices are preferable to a needle or blade, because the puncture depth is standardized.

4. Collect small blood specimens in the appropriate containers promptly after the procedure, and wipe the puncture site clean of excess blood.

5. Apply a dry, sterile gauze dressing until the bleeding stops.

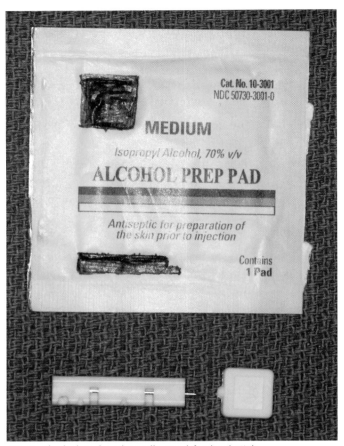

66-1 Alcohol pad and needle used for heel stick.

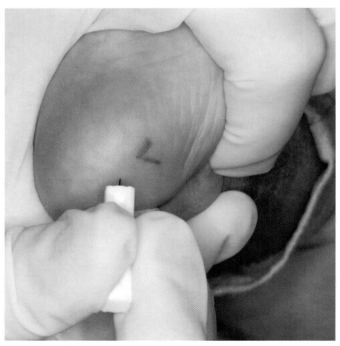

66-2 Puncture site for heel stick.

COMPLICATIONS:

- Osteochondritis of the calcaneous bone

- Infection of overlying skin and soft tissues

- Bruising

POST-PROCEDURE CARE:

1. No follow up is typically indicated.

2. In the infant receiving multiple heel sticks, sites should be rotated.

PEARLS/TIPS:

- Measurements of the hematocrit by heel stick in infants can be falsely elevated due to "milking" the site producing hemoconcentration. If polycythemia is suspected, a repeat measurement of the hematocrit should be obtained by peripheral venipuncture.

- Capillary blood gas values obtained by heel sticks may not accurately reflect arterial blood gas values.

67. Intraosseous Infusion

PURPOSE: To obtain rapid vascular access in children in whom regular vascular access is not obtainable for the purpose of administering fluid resuscitation, vasopressor therapy, anticonvulsants, or sodium bicarbonate.

EQUIPMENT NEEDED (FIGURE 67-1):

- Intraosseous needle (An 18- to 20-gauge spinal needle can be used in children less than 18 months of age; a 13- to 16-gauge bone marrow needle can be used in older children.)

- Povidone iodine (Betadine) solution

- 1% Lidocaine with 25-gauge needles and syringe (optional)

- 0.9% sodium chloride solution (physiologic saline)

- Intravenous tubing

- Three-way stopcock

- Intravenous fluids

- 20-cc syringe

- Tape

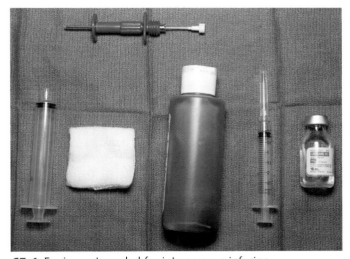

67-1 Equipment needed for intraosseous infusion.

- Padded board
- Pressure bag (if necessary)

TECHNIQUE:

IMPORTANT NOTE: Intraosseous vascular access should only be used as a temporary intravascular access in an emergency when conventional intravenous access cannot be obtained. The optimal needle insertion site for all ages is the anterior medial surface of the proximal tibia, approximately one finger breadth (2 to 3 cm) distal to the tibial tubercle (Figure 67-2). The distal femur, 3 to 4 cm above the external condyles, can also be used in small infants. Intravenous fluids may not flow by gravity through an intraosseous needle, necessitating the use of a pressure bag, particularly for rapid infusions.

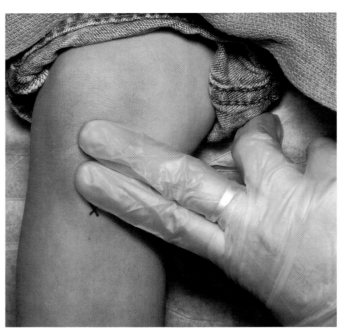

67-2 Optimal site for intraosseous infusion.

1. Clean the skin over the site thoroughly with a povidone-iodine solution.

2. Infiltrate the site with 1% lidocaine down to the periosteum, if time permits.

3. Insert the intraosseous needle at a slight angle (about 15 degrees) away from the growth plate until bony resistance is felt.

4. Advance the needle through the periosteum and into the bone using direct pressure with a twisting or screwing motion. A loss of resistance or a "pop" can be felt as the needle passes in to the marrow cavity.

5. Remove the stylet once the needle penetrates into the bone marrow, and attach a 20-cc syringe to the needle and attempt to aspirate some of the bone marrow. Aspiration of marrow confirms intraosseous needle placement, but in young infants bone marrow is often difficult to visualize. Rarely, bone marrow can occlude the needle.

6. Verify proper placement of the needle further by infusion of 5–10 mL of 0.9% sodium chloride solution through a syringe using gentle pressure with close observation for any extravasation of fluid.

7. Attach IV tubing to the intraosseous needle once the needle placement is confirmed, and administer intravenous fluids or medications.

8. Immobilize the utilized extremity with tape to a padded board. Most intraosseous needles have protective guards that can be secured with tape.

COMPLICATIONS:

- Extravasation of intravenous fluids into soft tissues due to improper placement of the intraosseous needle, with secondary soft tissue necrosis or compartment syndrome

- Osteomyelitis, cellulitis, or superficial infections

- Fracture or damage to the growth plate or epiphysis

- Fat embolus

POST-PROCEDURE CARE:

1. Immobilize the intraosseous needle and utilize extremity firmly to prevent dislodging. If a spinal needle is used, a hemostat can be attached to the needle and secured with tape.

2. Obtain placement of a more stable intravascular access as soon as possible.

PEARLS/TIPS:

- An intraosseous needle should be removed as soon as reliable vascular access is established elsewhere.

- In small infants, penetration of the needle through the entire bone can easily occur, resulting in puncture wounds to the holder or operator.

68. Lumbar Puncture in Infants and Small Children

PURPOSE: To obtain a sample of the cerebrospinal fluid (CSF) for bacteriologic, cellular, and chemical examination to evaluate for possible central nervous system infection, inflammation, or malignancy; to administer medications such as spinal anesthetics and antineoplastic agents; or to perform myelography.

EQUIPMENT NEEDED (FIGURE 68-1):

- Consent form

- Sterile gloves

- Spinal tap tray (infant, child, adult) includes: CSF specimen bottles, sterile drapes, spinal needles (20- to 22-gauge), disposable plastic manometer and stopcock, sponge applicators, local anesthetic, and syringe with fine needle for subcutaneous anesthetic administration

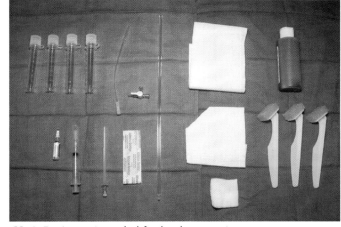

68-1 Equipment needed for lumbar puncture.

- Mask with face shield for eye protection
- Povidone iodine (Betadine) solution
- Sterile dressing and self-adhesive bandage

TECHNIQUE:

IMPORTANT NOTE: Before the procedure, the patient or guardian should be fully informed of the nature of the procedure and potential complications. A consent form should be signed by the patient or guardian and witnessed. Although the procedure can be performed alone, it is preferable to have an assistant who can hold the patient in the proper position. This is essential with young children and combative patients.

1. Perform the procedure on a firm surface (not in a hospital bed).

2. Place the patient in a lateral decubitus position, except in the neonate where the sitting position may be preferred (Figure 68-2).

3. Position the patient's lumbosacral area as close to the edge of the examination table as possible.

4. Have the patient curled up with the hands around the knees with the neck flexed forward. The knees should be as close to the chest as possible.

5. Put on sterile gloves.

6. Clean the lumbosacral region thoroughly with povidone iodine solution, spiraling outward from the lumbar spine, and allow to dry.

7. Lay a sterile drape with a fenestrated opening over the patient with the opening over the previously cleansed lumbar spine.

8. Approximate the L3-L4 vertebral inner space by placing the fingers of the nondominant hand on the anterior superior iliac crest while palpating the inner space with the thumb (Figure 68-3).

9. Perform the lumbar puncture only below the second lumbar vertebra, preferably between the L3-L4 inner space. A small amount of 1% lidocaine (0.2 mL) can be injected subcutaneously over the inner space for anesthesia.

10. Insert the needle exactly in the midline. A stylet should be inside the needle to minimize bleeding and introduction of skin fragments into the spinal canal (Figure 68-4). A change in resistance is typically noted as the needle penetrates the dura and enters the subarachnoid space, creating a palpable "pop."

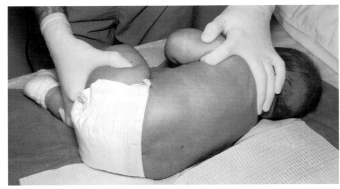

68-2 Lateral decubitus position for lumbar puncture.

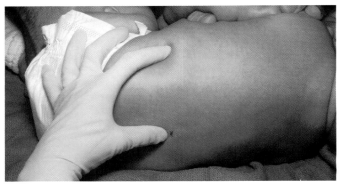

68-3 Palpating for the L3 to L4 vertebral innerspace.

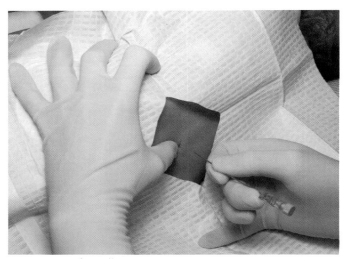

68-4 Point of needle insertion.

11. Remove the stylet to check for the flow of CSF (Figure 68-5). If no flow is noted, replace the stylet and advance the needle slightly before checking for CSF flow again.

12. Watch for blood flow through the spinal needle; this typically indicates that the needle has advanced into the posterior venous plexus in the spinal canal.

13. Measure the CSF opening pressure (if desired) using the manometer included in the spinal tap kit once CSF has begun to drip from the needle.

14. Collect 3 to 4 mL of cerebrospinal fluid in the supplied tubes (Figure 68-6).

15. Withdraw the needle.

16. Apply firm pressure to the puncture site for several minutes, after which apply an occlusive sterile dressing.

17. Send the labeled tubes of CSF for cell count with differential, glucose, protein, bacteriologic culture (viral, fungal, and acid-fast cultures can also be requested), and special stains. Gram stains are typically performed, but fungal, India ink, and acid-fast stains can be performed also, as needed. Additional studies such as VDRL, polymerase chain reaction (PCR), and latex-particle agglutination can be performed based on the patient's suspected diagnosis.

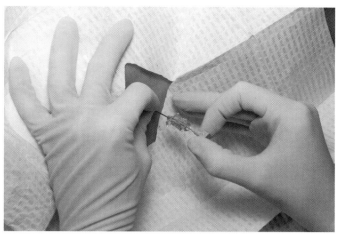

68-5 Removal of stylet.

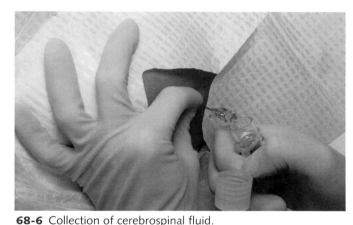

68-6 Collection of cerebrospinal fluid.

COMPLICATIONS:

- Localized infection at the lumbar puncture site

- Mild bruising or bleeding at the puncture site

- Local nerve damage

- Transient mild pain or discomfort at puncture site

- Headache

- An increased risk of fatal cerebellar or tentorial herniation in the presence of high central nervous system pressure

- Subdural or subarachnoid hemorrhage

POST-PROCEDURE CARE:

1. Minimize the risk of headache following lumbar puncture by having the patient remain in a reclined position.

PEARLS/TIPS:

- Contraindications include (lumbar puncture should *not* be attempted if the patient has):

  ◆ Cardiorespiratory instability

  ◆ Evidence of increased intracranial pressure (blurred optic discs, prominently bulging fontanelle)

  ◆ Local infection at the lumbar puncture site

- Uncorrected coagulation defects

- Concomitant measurement of blood glucose immediately before or after the lumbar puncture is essential to determine the CSF:blood glucose ratio.

- Aspiration of CSF from the spinal needle with a syringe should never be attempted.

- If viral meningoencephalitis is suspected, viral cultures of the CSF should be requested separately.

69. Umbilical Vein Catheterization

PURPOSE: Emergent vascular access for IV fluids or emergency medications in a neonate; long-term central venous access in neonates; central venous pressure monitoring.

EQUIPMENT NEEDED (FIGURE 69-1):

- Double-lumen umbilical vein catheters in appropriate sizes (No. 5F catheter for infants weighing less than 3.5 kg, No. 8F catheter for infants weighing more than 3.5 kg)

- Sterile drapes

- Sterile cap, gown, and gloves

- Umbilical tape

- Tape measure

- Povidone iodine (Betadine) swabs

- Two curved hemostats

- Two iris forceps with teeth

- Two straight forceps

- Needle driver

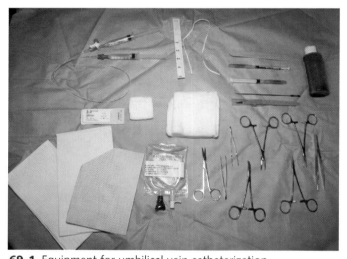

69-1 Equipment for umbilical vein catheterization.

- Suture scissors

- Silk suture

- Three-way stopcock

- Clave

- Two 3- or 5-mL syringes

- Flush solution

- Povidone iodine (Betadine)

- Good light source

Note: Some institutions have prepackaged umbilical vessel catheterization trays available for use.

TECHNIQUE:

1. Determine the appropriate depth of insertion. One easy method to determine the depth of insertion is to measure the distance from the shoulder to the umbilicus (in centimeters) and subtract 2 cm. The desired location of the catheter tip is 0.5 to 1.0 cm above the diaphragm. In this position, one can obtain central venous pressure monitoring. In emergent situations, a catheter can be advanced 3 cm or just until blood return is obtained and used for fluid or medication administration while avoiding hepatic infusion.

2. Prepare the catheter by placing the three-way stopcock and the clave on the end of each catheter lumen and filling the catheter with sterile saline flush solution.

3. Place the infant in a supine position, arrange a diaper over both thighs, and secure the infant by placing tape across the diaper-covered legs and the bed. This allows the feet to be visualized to monitor circulation for vasospasm. The upper extremities can be secured in a similar fashion.

4. Prepare the abdominal wall and umbilicus with povidone iodine using sterile technique.

5. Put on your sterile cap, gown, and gloves.

6. Use the sterile umbilical tape to tie the base of the umbilicus snugly, but not so tight that the catheter will not be able to pass through the vessel.

7. Cut the excess umbilical cord with a scalpel, leaving a 1-cm stump.

8. Identify the umbilical vein. There are normally two arteries and one vein. The arteries are thick-walled and often located at 4 o'clock and 7 o'clock. The vein is a thin-walled vessel located toward the periphery of the cord.

9. Grasp the end of the umbilicus with a curved hemostat and hold it steady. Open and dilate the umbilical vein with the curved iris forceps or the dilator included in the tray (Figure 69-2).

10. Insert the catheter when the vessel is sufficiently dilated, and advance slowly. You may grasp the catheter about 0.5 cm from the tip with the straight forceps to aid in insertion.

11. Check to see if there is blood return and that the catheter flushes easily.

12. Suture the catheter in place. First, take a single through-and-through stitch in the umbilical stump near the catheter and secure with a square knot. Remove the needle. Wrap the long segments of suture around the catheter and secure it with square knots; repeat this process a few times until the catheter is secure.

13. The catheter can then be secured additionally with tape (Figure 69-3).

COMPLICATIONS:

- Infection

- Thromboembolism

- Hepatic necrosis and portal hypertension—do not leave a catheter in the portal system.

- Cardiac arrhythmias can result from a catheter that has been inserted too far and is irritating the heart.

POST-PROCEDURE CARE:

1. Obtain an x-ray to confirm correct placement before using the catheter.

2. Never advance the catheter once the sterile field has been broken.

PEARLS/TIPS:

- If you encounter resistance or detect a "bobbing" motion of the catheter during insertion, the catheter may have entered the portal vein. To correct this you may try backing out and applying mild manual pressure in the right upper quadrant over the liver as you attempt to advance the catheter again.

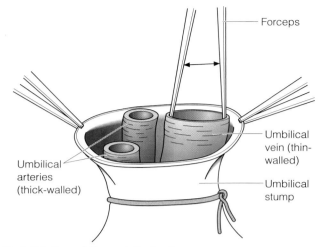

69-2 Dilation of the umbilical vein.

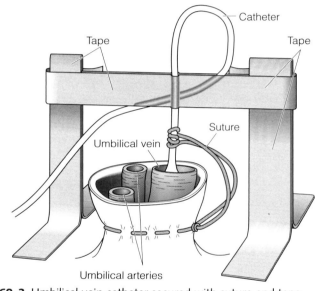

69-3 Umbilical vein catheter secured with suture and tape.

70. Nursemaid's Elbow Reduction

PURPOSE: To reduce subluxation of the radial head.

EQUIPMENT NEEDED:

- None

TECHNIQUE:

1. Supinate the forearm with the thumb over the radial head. A snap is often perceived as the radial head reduces (Figures 70-1a, 70-1b, 70-1c).

2. Flex the elbow if reduction is not successful. Some resistance may be noted as full flexion is approached. Gently pushing the elbow through the resistance will allow the annular ligament to slip back into normal position.

3. Instruct the patient (or parent or guardian) to begin using the extremity 10 to 15 minutes after the reduction is complete.

COMPLICATIONS:

- In children that present 1 to 2 days after the initial injury, there may be a longer delay between the time from reduction to resumption of full use of the extremity because of increased swelling of the annular ligament.

POST-PROCEDURE CARE:

1. Watch for resumption of normal use of the extremity after reduction.

2. Immobilization is not routinely recommended.

3. Counsel parents regarding the significant risk of recurrence with movements causing excessive traction on an extended elbow with forearm pronated.

PEARLS/TIPS:

- Some children, especially those who present later after the initial injury, will have some residual aching pain after the reduction. These children may benefit from acetaminophen for approximately 12 hours after reduction.

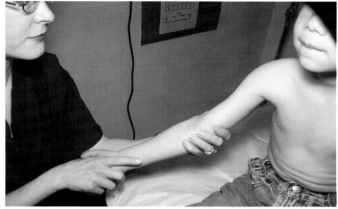

70-1a Motions for nursemaid's elbow reduction.

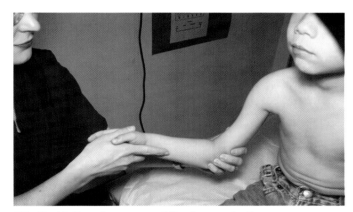

70-1b Motions for nursemaid's elbow reduction.

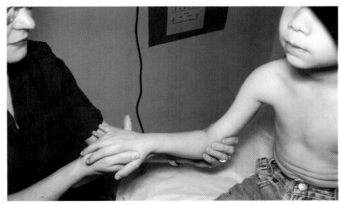

70-1c Motions for nursemaid's elbow reduction.

71. Male Circumcision

PURPOSE: Removal of foreskin from the penis in a newborn male.

EQUIPMENT NEEDED:

- 1-cc syringe with 30-gauge needle and 1% lidocaine without epinephrine for dorsal penile nerve block
- Three hemostats, at least one straight
- Sterile probe with a blunt tip
- Sterile scissors
- Safety pin (for Gomco circumcision)
- Scalpel

TECHNIQUE:

IMPORTANT NOTE: Prepare the foreskin before removal by breaking down adhesions and creating a dorsal slit as described in steps 1 through 6 below.

1. Inspect the penis and look for the urethral meatus; if it is malpositioned (i.e., hypospadias), then do not proceed.

2. Inject 0.5 cc of lidocaine without epinephrine subcutaneously at the 2 o'clock and 10 o'clock positions at the base of the penis. This is the dorsal penile nerve block.

3. Clamp two hemostats into place on either side of the apex of the foreskin on the dorsal surface.

4. Use the blunt end of the sterile probe, and in a vertical motion, probe from the apex of the foreskin to the base of the penis (keeping the tip of the probe in view). Break down as many of the adhesions as possible that attach the inner part of the foreskin to the penis. *Avoid breaking down the frenulum,* which is located on the ventral surface of the penis.

5. Take a straight pair of hemostats and, at the dorsal side of the penile foreskin, go 2/3 of the way down from the apex toward the corona and clamp the hemostats on the foreskin for approximately 60 seconds. This results in crush necrosis of the skin and will serve as the base for your dorsal slit. Use the sterile scissors and cut the length of the slit that you just used the hemostats to necrose.

6. Pull the foreskin down to expose the corona of the penis. Break down all adhesions using the blunt end of the probe or a 2 inch × 2 inch sterile gauze bandage. Once all the adhesions are broken down, you are ready to proceed with any of three methods of circumcision.

71a. Mogen

PURPOSE: Removal of foreskin from the penis in a newborn male.

EQUIPMENT NEEDED:

- Mogen clamp (Figure 71-1)
- No. 10 or 11 sterile disposable scalpel
- Gauze bandage

TECHNIQUE:

1. Follow steps 1 through 6 listed in "71. Male Circumcision" before performing the procedure.

2. Open the Mogen clamp fully, making sure that it opens no wider than 3 millimeters.

3. Push the glans back out of the way using the thumb and index finger, and pinch the foreskin below the dorsal hemostat.

4. Slide the Mogen clamp across the foreskin from dorsal to ventral, following along the same angle as the corona, and ensure that the apex of the dorsal slit is above the clamp.

5. Position the hollow side of the clamp facing the glans.

6. Make sure that the glans is free of the apparatus before shutting the clamp.

7. Keep the clamp in place for 1 1/2 minutes total, then use the scalpel to excise the foreskin.

8. Remove the clamp and gently but slowly separate the foreskin to expose the glans.

9. Use a gauze bandage to provide traction.

COMPLICATIONS:

- Bleeding
- Infection
- Need for revision of circumcision

POST-PROCEDURE CARE:

1. Place antibiotic ointment over the glans and then place the diaper back on the infant.

2. Document the next time that the infant voids or urinates.

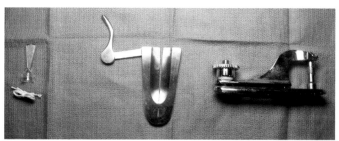

71-1 Different types of circumcision devices (from left to right): Plastibell, Gomco, Mogen.

PEARLS/TIPS:

• This technique is useful if there is no Gomco bell that comfortably fits over the glans of the penis.

71b. Gomco Clamp

PURPOSE: Removal of foreskin from the penis in a newborn male.

EQUIPMENT NEEDED:

• Gomco circumcision clamp (see Figure 71-1)

• Safety pin

• No. 10 or 11 sterile disposable scalpel

• 2 inch × 2 inch gauze bandage

TECHNIQUE:

IMPORTANT NOTE: The glans will vary in diameter and the Gomco bells are available in different sizes.

1. Follow steps 1 through 6 listed in "71. Male Circumcision" before performing procedure.

2. Ease the bell of the Gomco clamp into the space between the foreskin and the glans and cover the glans with the bell. The bell should be between the foreskin and the glans.

3. Secure the edges of the foreskin on either side of the dorsal slit with a safety pin to keep the bell from popping out of place.

4. Place the steel plate over the bell and gently pull the foreskin above the edge of the plate so that the end or apex of the dorsal slit is *above* the edge of the steel plate.

5. Clamp the apparatus in place using the stud.

6. Wait for 5 minutes to achieve as much crush necrosis of the foreskin as possible, thereby reducing the possibility of bleeding.

7. Use the sterile scalpel to excise the foreskin that is now above the edge of the plate. Remember, the glans is protected by the steel bell.

8. Take apart the Gomco apparatus once all of the foreskin is excised and the plate is completely exposed and clean.

9. Use a 2 inch × 2 inch gauze bandage to gently pull the edges of the foreskin away from the bell, and look for bleeding.

COMPLICATIONS:

- Bleeding

- Infection

- Need for revision of circumcision

POST-PROCEDURE CARE:

1. Place antibiotic ointment over the glans and then place the diaper back on the infant.

2. Document the next time that the infant voids or urinates.

PEARLS/TIPS:

- Make sure that the bell fits snugly over the glans of the penis; if it is too large, it can move around too easily when you are putting together the Gomco apparatus and can result in more bleeding.

71c. Plastibell

PURPOSE: Removal of foreskin from the penis in a newborn male.

EQUIPMENT NEEDED:

- Plastibell apparatus and string (see Figure 71-1)

TECHNIQUE:

IMPORTANT NOTE: Circumcision occurs through cutting off the blood supply to the distal foreskin using the string of the Plastibell.

1. Follow steps 1 through 6 listed in "71. Male Circumcision" before performing procedure.

2. Place the Plastibell device on the glans and pull the incised foreskin over it.

3. Bring the incised foreskin over the top of the Plastibell until the apex of the incision is above the string placement guide on the device (Figure 71-2).

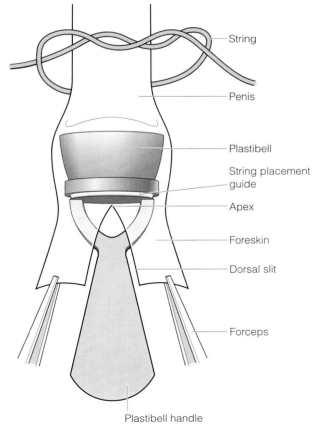

71-2 Circumcision: Plastibell placement.

4. Clamp the foreskin across the top of the Plastibell with a straight clamp (Figure 71-3).

5. Place the string around the foreskin and the Plastibell device in a groove so that it acts as the string placement guide.

6. Examine the area to make sure that the device has not slipped out of place and that the apex of the incision is distal to the placement of the string.

7. Tighten the string and tie it in a simple square knot. An adequate result is obtained when the skin just distal to the string blanches without the string breaking.

8. Trim the excess foreskin from around the bell using iris scissors (Figure 71-4).

9. Break the handle off the device.

COMPLICATIONS:

- Bleeding
- Infection
- Need for revision

POST-PROCEDURE CARE:

1. The remaining foreskin above the edge of the string will take 7 to 12 days to necrose and fall off.

PEARLS/TIPS:

- Educate the parents thoroughly about what to expect post-procedure, including the possibility that the infant may have redness and tenderness at site for up to 10 days.

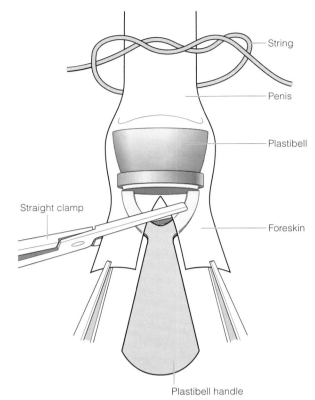

71-3 Circumcision: clamp across Plastibell.

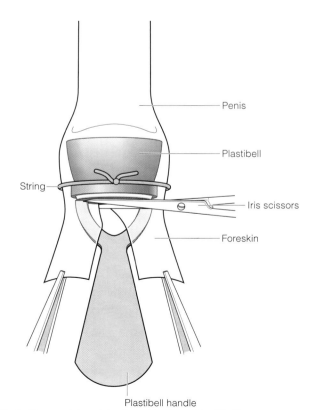

71-4 Circumcision: trim foreskin from Plastibell.

How to Interpret

(Figures A-1a and A1-b)

TECHNIQUE:

IMPORTANT NOTE: The technique for reading anteroposterior (AP), posteroanterior (PA), and lateral x-rays are the same (lateral films simply have more overlap of structures). In reading a chest x-ray it is very important to know your anatomy (especially the trachea, carina, aortic knob, heart, hilum, costophrenic angles, and stomach bubble) and to have a systematic approach. Do the same thing each time. You will come up with your own system fairly quickly, but until you do, use this one. Read each chest film in the following sequence: **A**bdomen, **T**horax, **M**ediastinum, **L**ungs (individually), **L**ungs (bilaterally). **ATMLL** can be remembered with the mnemonic **A**re **T**here **M**any **L**ung **L**esions?.

1. Look at the abdomen (area of least interest) below the diaphragm by scanning from the left upper quadrant across the abdomen. Look for the normal gas-containing structures such as the stomach, and splenic and hepatic flexures of the colon.

2. Scan the thorax (bone and soft tissue for now) by starting where your eyes left off in your abdominal scan (the right upper quadrant). Scan the bones and soft tissue of the right chest wall, up to the right shoulder, across to the left shoulder, and down to the left diaphragm angle. Do not miss these structures: right diaphragm angle, anterior and posterior ribs, breast tissue, scapula, clavicle, stomach, liver, and left diaphragm angle.

3. Examine the mediastinum. The mediastinum has many overlapping structures. Start your scan by looking for any widening. Next, look in more detail at the following structures: trachea, carina, aorta, heart, and hilum.

4. Look at the lungs individually. Start in the right diaphragm angle and work your way upward in a zigzag pattern looking at the right lung. For the left lung,

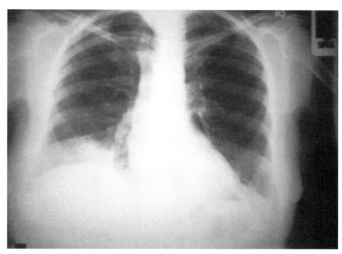

A-1a PA chest x-ray.

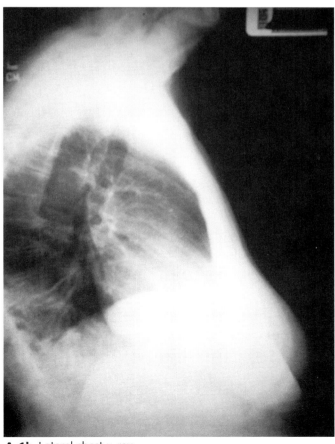

A-1b Lateral chest x-ray.

start at the left apex and zigzag down to the left diaphragm angle. During this lung scan, pay close attention to the lung tissue and any changes in density.

5. Look at the lungs bilaterally. Stand back and look at both lungs side by side for a comparison. By following this sequence each and every time you view a chest film, you will miss fewer findings.

PEARLS/TIPS:

- AP (anteroposterior, or portable) chest x-rays and PA chest x-rays are read as if the patient were standing in front of you facing your direction. Anterior ribs descend from lateral to medial, whereas posterior ribs descend from medial to lateral.

B. Abdominal X-ray Interpretation

(Figure B-1)

TECHNIQUE—BONES

Vertebral column

1. Look for all the landmarks—the pedicle, transverse process, spinous process, superior articulating process, lamina, and inferior articulating process.

2. Ensure that there is adequate space between vertebrae.

Lower ribs—Pelvis

1. Air in the cecum, sigmoid, and rectum and small bowel loops (if they contain air) will normally overlie the bones of the pelvis and sacrum.

2. On the AP view, identify the sacrum, ilium, ischium, pubis, obturator foramen, symphysis pubis, anterior superior iliac spine, acetabulum, femoral head, femoral neck, greater trochanter, lesser trochanter, and femoral shaft.

TECHNIQUE—SOFT TISSUES

Left upper quadrant

1. Look for the stomach; its air bubble helps to identify it.

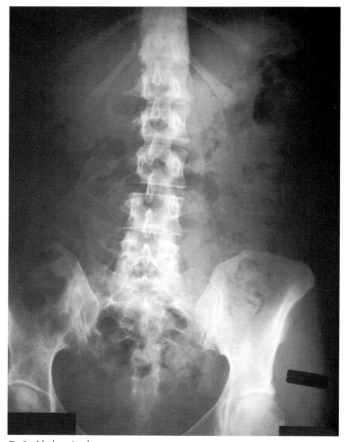

B-1 Abdominal x-ray.

2. Look for the shadow of the spleen.

3. Identify the splenic flexure; the position is variable.

Right upper quadrant

1. Look for the margin of the liver. The inferior limit of a gray mass or a boundary outlined by air in the transverse colon and hepatic flexure.

2. The shadow of the gallbladder may occasionally be visible as a rounded shadow superimposed on the liver margin and right kidney; only 15% of gallstones are calcified on plain films.

Both flanks

1. The upper poles of the kidneys are tilted toward the midline and against the psoas muscles; kidneys are usually partly obscured by varying amounts of gas and stool in the bowel.

2. The normal kidney length is 3.7 times the height of L2.

3. Look for the flank stripes (perirenal fat).

4. Look for the haustra of the large intestine.

Mid-abdomen

1. Follow the known course of the ureters along the psoas shadows to the bladder; look for any shadow that could represent a calculus; the ureters themselves are difficult to visualize without contrast material.

Pelvis

1. Check border indicators: organ masses, fat lines.

2. Look for calcification; shift in position, or change in shape of the structures.

TECHNIQUE—GASTROINTESTINAL (GI) TRACT

1. Look for the pattern of air or semisolid feces

C. Arterial Blood Gas Interpretation

PURPOSE: To determine the state of oxygenation and pH status of the patient. Once determinations are made, treatment can be started to correct the identified problems.

TECHNIQUE:

> IMPORTANT NOTE: Many factors can cause hypoxemic, acidemic, and alkalemic processes. Each is treated in a different fashion, which will not be discussed here. You should seek a text that discusses in detail respiratory and metabolic processes related to the oxygenation and pH status of patients.

1. Determine the state of oxygenation. Look at the pO_2. Is it less that 75 mm Hg? If so, the patient is hypoxemic.

2. Give the patient supplemental oxygen by the method most appropriate for his or her condition or situation, e.g., nasal cannula, Venturi mask, non-rebreather mask, continuous positive airway pressure/bilevel positive airway pressure (CPAP/BiPAP), or mechanical ventilator. The different types for the therapy methods appropriate to a given situation will not be discussed here.

3. Determine the pH status of the patient.

   a. If it is between 7.35 and 7.45, the pH is normal. There may be mild variations in the CO_2 and/or HCO_3 that will maintain the patient within this normal range.

   b. If it is below 7.35, the patient is considered to be acidemic. Next, determine if it is a respiratory or metabolic acidemia. If the CO_2 is high and the HCO_3 is normal, the patient suffers from respiratory acidemia. If the HCO_3 is low and the CO_2 is normal, the patient suffers from metabolic acidemia.

   c. If it is above 7.45, the patient is considered to be alkalemic. Next, determine if it is a respiratory or metabolic alkalemia. If the HCO_3 is high and the CO_2 is normal, the patient suffers from a metabolic alkalemia. If the CO_2 is low and the HCO_3 is normal, the patient suffers from a respiratory alkalemia.

PEARLS/TIPS:

- Normal arterial blood gas values:

pO_2	75 to 100 mm Hg
pCO_2	35 to 45 mm Hg
HCO_3	24 to 28 mEq/L
pH	7.35 to 7.45
% Saturation	90 to 100%

Appendices

A. Complete History and Physical Guidelines

HISTORY AND PHYSICAL

Primary information: List date, patient's name, and allergies.

Chief complaint (CC): Write CC in the patient's own words. For example, "I have chest pain."

History of present illness (HPI): Ask these questions about any pain: character, location, radiation, activities during onset, intensity, duration, alleviating or aggravating factors.

Past medical history (PMH): Ask about arthritis, asthma, hypertension, diabetes mellitus (DM), cancer, chronic obstructive pulmonary disease (COPD), heart disease, hepatitis, liver or kidney disease, rheumatic fever, seizures, tuberculosis (TB), thyroid disease, epilepsy, urinary tract infections (UTIs), and pneumonia.

Past surgical history (PSH): Ask whether the patient still has his or her gallbladder, appendix, or tonsils; patients often forget to mention these items.

Family medical history (FMH): The main diseases to inquire about are DM, hypertension, stroke, heart disease, cancer, and whether there are any inherited disorders.

Medications: List all current medications including prescription, over-the-counter, and herbal remedies.

Social history: Include patient's home location, size and composition of household, and occupation. Also record history of smoking (in pack-years), alcohol use (amount per day, type, how many years), and substance abuse

(illegal drugs). Cigarette pack-years = (packs per day) × (years spent smoking). Note: This information is often recorded as follows: *Patient is presently living in (city) with (household members) and works as a (occupation). Patient has history of (pack-years smoking), ETOH (drinks per day, type of alcohol, number of years), and substance abuse (illegal drugs).*

REVIEW OF SYSTEMS

a. Subject areas to discuss:

Review of systems (ROS): List any current symptoms, including pertinent positives and negatives (fever, nausea and vomiting, diarrhea or constipation, etc.). If patient complains of pain, ask about the following associated with the pain: location, quality, severity, timing (onset, duration, frequency), setting, aggravating or relieving factors, associated systems.

General: Recent weight change, fatigue, fever, sleep patterns, or insomnia

Skin: Rashes, lumps, sores, itching, dryness, color change, changes in hair or nails

HEENT

- **Head:** Headaches, head injury
- **Eyes:** Problems with vision; use of glasses or contact lenses; presence of pain, redness, glaucoma, cataracts
- **Ears:** Frequency of ear infections, loss of hearing
- **Nose and sinuses:** Frequent colds, nasal stuffiness, discharge, nosebleeds, sinus problems
- **Throat and mouth:** Frequent sore throats, hoarseness

Neck: Lumps in the neck, swollen glands, goiter, pain or stiffness in the neck

Breasts: Lumps, pain or discomfort, nipple discharge

Respiratory: Cough, sputum (color, quantity), hemoptysis, wheezing

Cardiac: High blood pressure, rheumatic fever, heart murmurs, chest pain or discomfort, palpitations, dyspnea, orthopnea, paroxysmal nocturnal dyspnea, edema, past ECG or other heart tests

Gastrointestinal (GI): Trouble swallowing, heartburn, appetite, nausea, vomiting of blood, indigestion. Bowel movements: color and size of stools, change in bowel habits, rectal bleeding or black tarry stools, hemorrhoids, constipation, diarrhea. Abdominal pain, liver or gallbladder problems, hepatitis

Urinary: Frequency of urination, polyuria, nocturia, burning or pain on urination, hematuria, urgency, reduced force of the urinary stream, hesitancy, incontinence, urinary infections, stones

Genital
- **Male:** Hernias, penile discharge or sores, testicular pain or masses, any sexually transmitted diseases (STDs) and their treatments
- **Female:** Age of menarche; regularity, frequency, and duration of periods; amount of bleeding, bleeding between periods or after intercourse, last menstrual period; dysmenorrhea; age at menopause, menopausal symptoms, postmenopausal bleeding. Discharge, itching, sores, lumps, any STDs and treatments. Number of pregnancies, number and type of deliveries, number of abortions (spontaneous and induced), complications of pregnancy, contraceptive methods

Peripheral vascular: Intermittent claudication, leg cramps, varicose veins, clots in the veins, Raynaud's disease (phenomenon)

Musculoskeletal: Muscle or joint pains, stiffness, arthritis, backache

Neurologic: Fainting, blackouts, seizures, weakness, paralysis, numbness, tingling, tremors, or other involuntary movements

Hematologic: Anemia, easy bruising or bleeding, past transfusions and possible reactions

Endocrine: Heat or cold intolerance, excessive sweating, excessive thirst or hunger, polyuria

Psychiatric: Mood including depression, any suicidal ideations, memory

b. Examples of how to write review of systems:

HEENT: *H*ead: Patient denies headaches. *E*yes: Patient denies any blurriness or vision changes. *E*ars: Patient denies ear pain or hearing changes. *N*ose: No discharge. *T*hroat: Patient denies a sore throat or mouth lesions.

Respiratory: *Patient denies shortness of breath, cough, or wheezing.* (If patient has respiratory disease, ask if patient uses oxygen at home and if so, how much and how often.)

Cardiovascular: *Patient denies chest pain, shortness of breath, palpitations, orthopnea, or paroxysmal nocturnal dyspnea.*

GI: *Patient denies diarrhea, constipation, nausea, vomiting, melena, or bright red blood per rectum.*

Genitourinary (GU): *No dysuria, frequency, or hesitancy.*

Neurologic: *Patient denies any numbness or tingling in extremities.*

PHYSICAL EXAM (including examples of how to write the information gathered):

Vital Signs: Record temperature, heart rate, respiratory rate, blood pressure, height, and weight.

General: *This is a (##) year old (male/female) who appears well-hydrated and properly nourished, and whose appearance is appropriate with the stated age. The patient is alert, cooperative, and in no acute distress at this time.*

Skin: *Skin texture, turgor, and pigmentation appear normal. No rashes.*

Head: *NCAT, symmetrical and without deformities.* (**NCAT: n**ormo**c**ephalic, **at**raumatic.)

Eyes: *PERRLA/EOMI bilaterally.* (**PERRLA: p**upils **e**qual **r**ound and **r**eactive to **l**ight and **a**ccommodation; **EOMI: e**xtraocular **m**otion **i**ntact.)

Ears: *External ear canals patent. TMs intact bilaterally with normal cone of light without injection.* (**TM: t**ympanic **m**embrane.)

Nose: *No septal deviation, turbinates appear (normal/pink) without hyperemia or exudates.*

Throat and mouth: *Oropharynx (pink/moist). Clear without hyperemia or lesions. (Good/poor) dentition.*

Neck: *Carotid pulses equal (2+). No carotid bruits. No cervical lymphadenopathy.*

Lungs: *Lungs clear to auscultation bilaterally. No (wheezes/rales/crackles/rhonchi).*

Cardiac: *Regular rate and rhythm without (murmur/ gallop/rub). JVP (##) cm above the right atrium.*

Breasts: *Breasts are symmetrical; no skin changes; no nipple discharge; no lumps or masses palpated.* (Don't forget to palpate axilla, as breast tissue extends into this region.)

Abdomen: *Normal active bowel sounds. No masses, organomegaly, or rebound tenderness. No costovertebral tenderness. No TTP.* If there is tenderness to palpation (TTP), note location, quality, etc.

Extremities: *No clubbing, cyanosis, or edema. Bilateral DP and posterior tibial PT pulses palpable. Calves supple without tenderness.* It is important to check on inpatients because of possible deep venous thrombosis (DVT) formation from lying supine for extended periods of time. **DP: d**orsalis **p**edis; **PT: p**osterior **t**ibial.

Neurologic: *Patient oriented × 3 (to person, place, time). Deep tendon reflexes (DTRs) equal and adequate (2/4) in biceps, patellar tendons. Motor 5/5 in upper and lower extremities. Normal gait, negative Romberg, normal finger to nose. Cranial nerves II through XII grossly intact.* Note fine hand tremor when hands extended outward for alcoholic patients, could signify beginning of delirium tremens (DTs). If patient indicates dizziness or fainting, obtain orthostatics, which include blood pressure and pulse in supine, sitting, and standing positions. If more than 20 point change in pulse or systolic pressure with sitting or standing, the patient is positive and hemodynamically unstable.

- Cranial nerve I: Smell

- Cranial nerve II: Vision and visual fields

- Cranial nerves III, IV, VI: Pupillary light response, extraocular eye movements, ptosis

- Cranial nerve V: Sensory portion is facial sensation, corneal reflex; motor portion is jaw opens against resistance

- Cranial nerve VII: Smile, close eyes tightly (practitioner should not be able to open them), wrinkle forehead, puff out cheeks

- Cranial nerve VIII: Hearing (tuning fork tests and whisper test)

- Cranial nerves IX, X: Speech; when patient says "ah" there should be equal and upward motion of palette

- Cranial nerve XI: Patient can turn head against resistance and shrug shoulders

- Cranial nerve XII: Patient can stick out tongue midline with no deviation to either side

Rectal: *Normal sphincter tone. No masses, polyps, hemorrhoids palpated. No gross blood noted. Stool brown and hemoccult (positive/negative). Prostate without nodules and non-tender to palpation nor enlarged* (or state *"deferred at this time"*).

GU, male: *Normal. No discharge, inflammation, or evidence of infection. Testes descended, no palpable nodules.*

GU, female: *Normal female external genitalia, vaginal mucosa moist, pink. Cervix visualized. Pap smear obtained. Uterus is normal size (usually noted as 6 week* *size) and in (ante/retro) position. Bimanual exam revealed no adenexal tenderness or masses. No cervical tenderness.*

Laboratory: Include complete blood count, comprehensive metabolic panel, basic metabolic panel, urinalysis, chest x-ray, cat scan, magnetic resonance imaging results, cardiac enzymes, etc.

Impressions: State problem list and plans here. For example:

- Problem: Patient condition (stable/fair/good/improving/worsening); lab tests or symptoms to give reason for patient condition assessment (*pt complains of SOB*); plan to correct or diagnose problem; etc.

- List as many as necessary; this also helps to organize your thoughts when you present your patient to the resident or attending.

- Go in order: Start with acute conditions then list chronic conditions (then list health maintenance items if in a primary care outpatient setting).

B. Progress and Procedure Note Samples

Always record the date and time (either military or conventional with AM/PM noted) on all notes and pages. Sign all notes legibly. Many of these notes are taken in the "SOAP" format (Subjective, Objective, Assessment, and Plan).

FAMILY AND INTERNAL MEDICINE PROGRESS NOTE:

- Record all IV fluids, medications and dosages in the margin.

- Record hospital day #, antibiotic and day #.

S: Any patient complaints or comments including: pain (location, intensity, duration), nausea, vomiting, bowel movements, urinary symptoms, appetite, chest pain, shortness of breath, and ambulation. Also include any nursing comments here.

O: Vital signs: Temperature, heart rate, respiratory rate, blood pressure, weight, and O_2 saturations (96% on 2 L via face mask or nasal cannula).

Ins/outs: IV fluids, by mouth (PO) intake, urine, bowel movements, emesis, drains

Physical exam: Including pulmonary with ventilator settings, as appropriate

Cardiovascular: Telemetry for past 24 hours, as appropriate

Results of labs, procedures, and radiologic findings (most recent findings; also have previous day's lab results available)

A: For each assessment, note patient's condition and reason.

P: Plan for each problem noted. Include as needed: medication or IV fluid changes; diet and ambulation changes; discontinuing Foley catheter, drains, or patient-controlled analgesia (PCA) pump; labs or procedures; consults and discharge plans.

SURGERY PROGRESS NOTE:

- Record all IV fluids, medications and dosages in the margin.

- Record hospital day number, post-op day number, antibiotic and day number.

S: Patient complains of (complaint). Pt nothing by mouth (NPO) or tolerating (clears, full liquids, regular diet). Pain is well controlled on (medication). Note the following: voiding, flatus, bowel movements, nausea, vomiting, chest pain, shortness of breath, ambulation.

O: Vital signs: Temperature, heart rate, respiratory rate, blood pressure, weight, and O_2 saturations (96% on 2 liters via nasal cannula).

Ins/outs: IV fluids, oral (PO) intake, urine, bowel movements, emesis, drains (nasogastric tube [NGT], Foley, JP)

Physical exam: Include incision, noting clean, dry, intact, no erythema

Labs, procedures, and radiologic findings

A: Note patient's condition and reasoning for each assessment.

P: Plan for each problem noted. Include as needed: medication or IV fluid changes; diet and ambulation changes; incentive spirometry; discontinuing Foley catheter, drains, or PCA pump; labs or procedures; consults (physical therapy [PT], respiratory therapy [RT], social services) and discharge plans.

OBSTETRICS NOTES

Obstetrics Admit Note:

- ID: (Age) year old G_ P_ at (gestation in weeks) weeks by last menstrual period and ultrasound (record dates). (Gravida—number of pregnancies, Para—number carried to term or live children.)

- CC: Onset of contractions, loss of fluid, fetal movement, vaginal bleeding.

- HPI: Prenatal care (location and beginning date), ultrasound results, group B streptococcal (GBS) status, rubella immunity, Rh positive/negative.

- Past medical, surgical, and OB history: Include recent Pap smear results.

- Allergies: Don't forget latex!

- Social: Tobacco, alcohol, drug use

- Physical Exam: Also record additional OB exam, including palpable contractions, position (vertex), fetal heart tones, frequency of contractions, standard vaginal exam (dilation, effacement, station), edema, and deep tendon reflexes.

- Assessment: Active labor, any pertinent findings (GBS+), desires epidural.

- Plan: Include if needed: amniotomy, augmentation, epidural, and medications.

Obstetrics Progress Note for Labor and Delivery Patients:

- Usually taken every 2 hours.

S: Pain control. Need to push. Amniotomy performed, with/without meconium staining.

O: Vital signs, fetal heart tones (presence of fetal scalp electrode [FSE]; include rate; comment on beat-to-beat variability and presence of accelerations or decelerations), frequency of contractions (whether external or internal uterine contractions are being monitored and recorded), standard vaginal exam (dilation, effacement, station)

A: (Age) year old G_P_ at (gestation in weeks) weeks in active labor. Note presence of meconium staining.

P: Augmentation if necessary; expect delivery soon. (Increase in pitocin dose, etc.)

Obstetrics Delivery Note:

Pt is a (age) year old G_P_ at (gestation in weeks) weeks' gestation. Pt delivered a live born male/female infant at (time, date) by (spontaneous vaginal delivery, classic c-section) to a sterile field. Anesthesia: (none, local, pudendal, epidural). Infant was (bulb, DeLee) suctioned on the perineum and handed to nursing staff. Apgars were (score) and (score) at 1 and 5 minutes, weight of (weight) grams. Infant sent to newborn nursery stable. Placenta (spontaneously, manually) delivered at (time), intact with a three-vessel cord. Cord blood sent to lab. (Degree laceration, episiotomy, incision) repaired with (name of suture) suture (3-0 Vicryl) in usual fashion. Estimated blood loss: (volume) cc. Mother sent to postpartum ward stable. Note names of all physicians in attendance.

Postpartum Progress Note:

S: Pt complaints or comments. Include: pain control, amount of vaginal bleeding, tolerating diet, flatus, bowel movements, urination, nausea, vomiting, breast tenderness, breast/bottle feeding, birth control plans, ambulation.

O: Vital signs, physical exam

Fundal height, firmness

Laceration repair, incision, episiotomy clean, dry, intact, no erythema.

A: Pt is a (age) year old G_P_ status post (standard vaginal delivery, c-section). Postpartum day (number).

P: Continue routine postpartum care. Medications or IV fluid changes, labs, encourage ambulation, advance diet, discharge plans.

Postpartum Discharge Orders:

- Diagnosis: (Spontaneous vaginal delivery, c-section) at (gestation in weeks) weeks

- Other: Abnormal Pap smear results, DM, placental complications

- Procedures: Laceration repair, bilateral tubal ligation, etc.

- Instructions: Pelvic rest for 6 weeks; no driving/heavy lifting for 2 weeks; call or return if experience temperatures above 101°F, persistent nausea or vomiting, increased vaginal bleeding or abdominal pain, or any other problems or concerns; use an infant car seat; no smoking around baby.

- Discharge meds: Laxative, Tylenol, prenatal vitamins, iron, birth control

- Diet: Regular, or ADA

- Activity: As above

NEWBORN NOTES

Newborn Admission Note:

- Pt is a (age) week (appropriate for gestational age [AGA], large for gestational age [LGA], small for gestational age [SGA]) male/female status post (standard vaginal delivery [SVD], or c-section secondary to (repeat, breech, or fetal intolerance to labor). Pt born to a (age) year old G_P_ mother.

- Mother's labs: Blood type, Rh status, HIV status, HbsAg status, rubella immunity, GBS status, *Chlamydia* and gonorrhea status.

- Prenatal care: None, limited, or early

- Complications with pregnancy: Substance abuse, infections, pre-eclampsia, DM, medications

- Rupture of membranes: (Hours) hours prior to delivery; clear, thick meconium, blood

- Complications with delivery: Fetal heart rate decelerations, vacuum, forceps, breech presentation, intrapartum meds

- Resuscitation: Include Apgar scores at 1 and 5 minutes of life

- Birth weight: (Weight) grams; length: (length) cm; fronto-occipital circumference (FOC): (measurement) cm

Physical exam

- Labs: Blood type, Coombs, and RPR

- Assessment: Example: Pt is a term AGA male status post SVD to a 22-year-old G2P2 mother, doing well.

- Plan: Admit to newborn nursery. Routine care and instructions. Continue breastfeeding/formula ad lib. Mother does/does not want circumcision.

Newborn Discharge Note:

- Diagnosis: Term AGA male/female

- Procedures: Hepatitis B No. 1 vaccine (date); newborn screen; hearing screen; circumcision

- Instructions: Keep all future appointments; use car seat; no smoking around infant; alcohol to umbilical cord daily; call or return if temperature over 100.4°F,

increased emesis, decreased PO intake, increased loose stools, or any other problems or concerns.

ADMIT ORDERS/TRANSFER ORDERS:

- Admit/Transfer: Floor, service (include resident and attending); telemetry

- Diagnosis: List in order of importance.

- Condition: Good, stable, critical

- Vitals: Per routine; every 4 hours

- Activity: Bed rest; out of bed to chair; ambulate with assistance 3× per day

- Allergies: No known drug allergies (NKDA); record reaction to allergy

- Nursing: I/Os routine, Foley to gravity, fall or seizure precautions, ted hose (support hose) incentive spirometry to bedside, accuchecks qAC (before meals) and before bedtime (qhs) for patients with diabetes, etc.

- Diet: NPO, clear liquid, full liquid, regular, American Diabetic Association (ADA), American Heart Association (AHA)

- IV fluids: (Type) at (volume) cc/hour with (concentration) mEq KCl/L.

- Medications: Include if needed: prn (as needed) meds, pain meds, sliding scale for administration of insulin, O_2 to maintain O_2 sats above (saturation percent) %.

- Labs: CBCD, BMP, ABG, ECG, x-rays, pulse oximetry, etc., as needed.

- Other: Respiratory care plan, social services consult

- Notify house officer on arrival.

PRE-OP NOTE:

- Pre-op diagnosis: List in order of importance

- Allergies: Note allergies; don't forget latex!

- Procedure: Surgery scheduled

- Labs: Record results

- Chest x-ray: Record results

- ECG: Record results

- Orders: Pt received pre-op antibiotics; pt nothing by mouth (NPO) after midnight

- Consent: Risks and benefits discussed, questions encouraged and answered. Pt agreed to procedure. Signed consent form in chart.

PROCEDURE NOTE:

- Procedure: (Procedure name)

- Indication/diagnosis: (Indication or diagnosis leading to procedure)

- Requiring: (Procedure)

- Consent: Risks and benefits discussed, questions encouraged and answered. Pt agreed to procedure. Signed consent form in chart.

- Physicians: Attending, residents, students

- Description of procedure: (Location of procedure). Area was prepped with (Betadine, Hibiclens) and draped in a sterile manner. Anesthetic: (volume) cc of (medication). Describe procedure; include type of instruments used, anatomic approach, and findings. Estimated blood loss (volume). Pt tolerated procedure (well, poorly).

- Complications: Unable to perform procedure due to (reason). Pt required CPR, etc.

- Labs/x-rays: Any labs or x-rays pertinent to procedure.

CENTRAL LINE PLACEMENT PROCEDURE NOTE:

- Indication: Record indication or diagnosis.

- Consent: Risks and benefits discussed, questions encouraged and answered. Pt agreed to procedure. Signed consent form in chart.

- Procedure: (Location of procedure). Type of catheter: (catheter name). Area was prepped with (Betadine/Hibiclens) and draped in a sterile fashion. Local anesthetic (volume) cc of (medication) was used. By sterile Seldinger technique, the (right/left) (vein name) vein was cannulated. A dilator was placed over the guide wire and the skin was successfully dilated. A scalpel (was/was not) required to incise the skin for the dilator to pass. The dilator was removed and a (single/multiple) lumen central line catheter was placed over the guide wire. The catheter was inserted into the vein to (distance) cm. Next, the guide wire was removed. Blood was drawn from all ports. The ports were then flushed with saline (with/without) heparin. The central line catheter was sutured to the skin with (suture).

- X-ray findings: Record findings.

- Complications: Note complications.

- Physicians: Attending, residents, students

INTUBATION PROCEDURE NOTE:

- Indication: List indication or diagnosis.

- Consent: Risks and benefits discussed, questions encouraged and answered. Pt agreed to procedure. Signed consent form in chart.

- Vital signs: Record vitals

- Maximum O_2 saturation pre-intubation: Record saturation.

- Procedure: Patient was oxygenated using bag valve mask with 100% O_2. Patient was sedated with (amount) mg of (medication), and induced with (amount) mg of (medication). Muscle relaxation was achieved with (amount) mg of (medication). Next, the patient was placed into the sniffing position and intubated with a size (size) Mac/Miller blade. Endotracheal tube size (size) mm was used and the cuff inflated. Breath sounds after intubation were (equal/unequal bilaterally). The endotracheal tube was secured at the lips/teeth at (distance) cm. An end tidal CO_2 detector (was/was not) used. ABG and CXR were ordered. The patient tolerated the procedure (well/poorly).

- Ventilator settings: Mode: SIMV/AC; tidal volume: (volume); FIO_2: (percent) %; PEEP: (pressure).

- Labs, chest x-ray results, and arterial blood gas (ABG) results: Record results.

- Complications: Note complications.

- Physicians: Attending, residents, students

DISCHARGE NOTE:

- Admission and discharge dates: Record dates.

- Admission and discharge diagnoses: List in order of importance.

- Physicians: Attending and residents

- Condition on discharge: Good, stable

- Discharge to: Home, nursing home, etc.

- Consults: Record.

- Procedures: Include date and results.

- Summary of admission history and physical: *Pertinent* findings

- Hospital course: Brief summary of findings and treatments

- Instructions: Keep all follow-up appointments. Take all medications as prescribed. Call physician, return to clinic, or go to ER if (complication specific to individual diagnosis) or any other problems or concerns.

• Medications: Medication names, dosages, frequency of administration, number of pills, and number of refills.

• Diet: Regular, ADA, AHA

• Activity: As tolerated; bed rest; with precautions

• Follow-up plans: Date and time of appointment with physician's name and location.

C. English-Spanish History and Physical Terms and Phrases

English	Spanish	Phonetic Spanish
I am the doctor (male).	Yo soy el doctor.	Yoh soh-ee ehl dohk-tohr.
I am the doctor (female).	Yo soy la doctora.	Yoh soh-ee lah dohk-tohr-ah.
My name is . . .	Me llamo . . .	Meh yah-moh . . .
I am going to ask you questions.	Voy a hacerle preguntas.	Boy ah ah-sehr-leh preh-goon-tahs.
When answering, please speak slowly.	Cuándo conteste, por favor hable despacio.	Kwahn-doh kohn-tehs-teh, pohr fah-vohr ah-bleh dehs-pah-see-oh.
I speak only a little Spanish.	Hablo solo un poquito de Español.	Ah-bloh soh-loh oon poh-kee-toh deh Ehs-pah-nyohl.
Please answer yes or no to the following questions.	Por favor conteste si o no a las siguientes preguntas.	Pohr-fah-vohr kohn-tehs-teh see oh noh ah lahs see-gee-ehn-tehs preh-goon-tahs.
Do you speak English?	Habla Inglés?	Ah-blah Een-glehs?
Is there anyone with you who speaks English?	Hay alguien con usted que hable Inglés?	Eye ahl-gee-ehn kohn oos-tehd keh ah-bleh Een-glehs?
What is your name?	Cómo se llama?	Koh-moh seh yah-mah?
How old are you?	Cuántos años tiene?	Koo-ahn-tohs ah-nyohs tee-eh-neh?
Please count on your fingers.	Por favor cuente en sus dedos.	Pohr fah-vohr kwehn-teh ehn soos deh-dohs

HPI: Always ask these about any pain: character, location, radiation, activities during onset, intensity, duration, alleviating or aggravating factors.

English	Spanish	Phonetic Spanish
Do you have pain?	Tiene dolor?	Tee-eh-neh doh-lohr?
Point with your finger where it hurts the most.	Señale con un dedo dónde le duele más.	Seh-nyah-leh kon oon deh-doh dohn-deh leh dweh-leh mas.
Is the pain . . .	Es el dolor . . .	Ehs ehl doh-lohr . . .
Constant?	Constante?	Constante?
Intermittent?	Intermitente?	Een-tehr-mee-tehn-teh?
Sharp?	Afilado?	Ah-fee-lah-doh?
Dull?	Monótono?	Moh-noh-toh-noh?
Burning?	Ardiente?	Ahr-dee-ehn-teh?
Cramping?	Retortijante?	Reh-tohr-tee-hohn-teh?
Squeezing?	Apretante?	Ah-preh-than-teh?
Throbbing?	Pulsante?	Pool-sahn-teh?
Aching?	Doloroso?	Doh-loh-roh-soh?
Mild?	Ligero?	Lee-heh-roh?
Moderate?	Moderado?	Moh-deh-rah-doh?
Severe?	Severo?	Seh-veh-roh?
Do you get the pain after meals?	Le da a usted el dolor después de comer?	Leh doh ah oos-tehd ehl doh-lohr dehs-pwehs deh koh-mehr?
Do you get the pain before meals?	Le da a usted el dolor antes de comer?	Leh doh ah oos-tehd ehl doh-lohr ahn-tehs deh koh-mehr?
Is the pain worse when breathing?	Es peor el dolor cuándo respira?	Ehs peh-ohr ehl doh-lohr kwahn-doh rehs-pee-rah
Is the pain worse when exerting yourself?	Es peor el dolor cuándo hace esfuerzo por si mismo?	Ehs peh-ohr ehl doh-lohr kwahn-doh ah-seh ehs-fwehr-soh pohr see mees-moh?

English	Spanish	Phonetic Spanish
Does the pain spread?	Se extiende el dolor?	*Seh egs-tee-ehn-deh ehl doh-lohr?*
Where?	Dónde?	*Dohn-deh?*
Does anything make it feel better?	Hay algo que lo hace sentir mejor?	*Eye ahl-goh keh loh ah-she sehn-teer meh-hohr?*
Does anything make it feel worse?	Hay algo que lo hace sentir peor?	*Eye ahl-goh keh loh ah-she sehn-teer peh-ohr?*
How many hours (days, weeks, months) has it been this way?	Cuántas horas (días, semanas, meces) hace de dolerle?	*Kwahn-tahs oh-rahs (dee-ahs, seh-mah-nahs, meh-ses) ah-seh deh doh-lehr-leh?*
Have you taken any medication for the pain?	Ha tomado alguna medicina para el dolor?	*Ah toh-mah-doh ahl-goo-nah meh-dee-see-nah pah-rah el doh-lohr?*
Please show me the medicine?	Por favor enseñeme la medicina?	*Pohr fah-vohr ehn-seh-nyeh-meh medicina?*
Are you having any . . .	Tiene usted alguna (algún) . . . (for bleeding use algún istead of alguna)	*Tee-eh-neh oos-tehd ahl-goo-nah (ahl-goon) . . .*
Bleeding?	Desangre?	*Deh-sahn-greh?*
Cough?	Tos?	*Tohs?*
Fever?	Fiebre?	*Fee-eh-breh?*
Diarrhea?	Diarrea?	*Dee-ah-rheh-ah?*
Dizzy spells?	Mareos?	*Mah-reh-ohs?*
Problem breathing?	Problema al respirar?	*Proh-bleh-mah ahl rehs-pee-rahr?*

PMH: Ask about arthritis, asthma, hypertension, diabetes, cancer, COPD/emphysema, heart disease, hepatitis, liver or kidney disease, rheumatic fever, seizures, tuberculosis, thyroid disease, epilepsy, urinary tract infections, and pneumonia. Allergies.

English	Spanish	Phonetic Spanish
Have you ever had . . .	Ha tenido usted . . .	*Ah teh-nee-doh oos-ted . . .*
Arthritis?	Artritis?	*Are-treeh-tees?*
Asthma?	Asma?	*Ahs-mah?*
Hypertension?	Presión alta?	*Preh-see-ohn ahl-tah?*
Diabetes?	Diabetes?	*Dee-ah-beh-tehs?*
Cancer?	Cáncer?	*Kehn-sehr?*
Emphysema?	Enfisema?	*Ehn-fee-seh-mah?*
Heart disease?	Enfermedad del corazón?	*Ehn-fehr-meh-dad dehl koh-rah-sohn?*
Hepatitis?	Hepatitis?	*Eh-pah-tee-tees?*
Liver problem?	Problema de higado?	*Proh-bleh-mah deh ee-gah-doh?*
Kidney problem?	Problema de riñon?	*Proh-bleh-mah deh ree-nyohn?*
Rheumatic fever?	Fiebre Reumática?	*Fee-eh-breh reh-oo-mah-tee-kah?*
Seizures?	Ataques epilépticos?	*Ah-tah-kehs eh-pee-lep-tee-kohs?*
Tuberculosis?	Tuberculosis?	*Too-behr-koo-loh-sees?*
Thyroid problem?	Problema de tiroide?	*Proh-bleh-mah deh tee-roy-deh?*
Urinary tract infections?	Una infección en la vehiga?	*Oo-nah een-feg-see-ohn ehn lah veh-hee-gah?*
Pneumonia?	Neumonia?	*Neh-oo-moh-nee-ah?*
Do you have allergies?	Tiene alergias?	*Tee-eh-neh ah-lehr-hee-ahs?*

PSH: Include here any significant surgeries. Always ask patients if they still have their gallbladder, appendix, or tonsils, because patients often forget about these.

English	Spanish	Phonetic Spanish
Have you had surgeries?	Ha tenido operaciones?	*Ah teh-nee-doh oh-peh-rah-see-ohn-ehs?*
Do you have your . . .	Tiene . . .	*Tee-eh-neh . . .*
Gallbladder?	Vesícula biliar?	*Veh-see-koo-lah bee-lee-ahr?*
Appendix?	Apéndice?	*Ah-pehn-dee-seh?*
Tonsils?	Tonsilas?	*Ton-see-las?*

FMH: The main diseases to inquire about are diabetes, heart disease, cancer, and whether there are any inherited disorders.

English	Spanish	Phonetic Spanish
Have any of your relatives had . . .	Alguno de sus parientes ha tenido . . .	*Ahl-goo-noh deh soos pah-ree-ehn-tehs ah teh-nee-doh . . .*
Diabetes?	Diabetes?	*Dee-ah-beh-tehs?*
Heart disease?	Enfermedad del corazón?	*Ehn-fehr-meh-dad dehl koh-rah-sohn?*
Cancer?	Cáncer?	*Kehn-sehr?*

MEDICATIONS: List all current medications including prescription, over-the-counter, and herbal remedies.

English	Spanish	Phonetic Spanish
Do you take any medicines?	Toma algunas medicinas?	*Toh-mah ahl-goo-nahs meh-dee-see-nahs?*
What medicines do you take?	Qué medicinas toma?	*Keh meh-dee-see-nahs toma?*

SOCIAL HISTORY: Patient is presently living in (city) with (household members) and works as a (occupation). Patient has history of (pack-years) for (number) years; ETOH (amount of alcohol per day, type of alcohol, and how many years), and substance abuse (illegal drugs). **Pack years of cigarettes = (No. of packs per day) × (No. of years spent smoking)

English	Spanish	Phonetic Spanish
Husband?	Esposo?	*Ehs-poh-soh?*
Wife?	Esposa?	*Ehs-poh-sah?*
Children?	Hijos?	*Ee-hohs?*
Do you drink alcohol?	Toma bebidas alcohólicas?	*Toh-mah beh-bee-dahs ahl-koh-lee-kahs?*
How many drinks/beers do you drink daily?	Cuántos tragos o cervezas se toma diario?	*Kwahn-tohs trah-gohs oh ser-veh-sahs seh toh-mah dee-ah-ree-oh?*
Do you smoke?	Fuma usted?	*Foo-mah oos-tehd?*
How many cigarettes per day?	Cuántos cigarillos por día?	*Koo-ahn-tohs see-gah-ree-yohs pohr dee-ah?*

English	Spanish	Phonetic Spanish
Show me with your fingers how many.	Enséñeme con sus dedos cuántos.	*Ehn-seh-nyeh-meh kohn soos deh-dohs kwahn-tohs.*
Are you employed?	Está usted empleado?	*Ehs-tah oos-tehd ehm-pleh-ah-doh?*
Do you use drugs?	Usa usted drogas?	*Oo-sah oos-tehd droh-gahs?*

REVIEW OF SYSTEMS

ROS: List any current symptoms including pertinent positives and negatives (fever, nausea and vomiting, diarrhea or constipation, etc.). If patient complains of pain, ask about the following associated with the pain: location, quality, severity, timing (onset, duration, frequency), setting, aggravating or relieving factors, associated systems.

English	Spanish	Phonetic Spanish
General:		
Gained weight lately?	Ha subido de peso últimamente?	*Ah soo-bee-doh deh peh-soh ool-tee-mah-mehn-teh?*
Fatigue?	Fatiga?	*Fah-tee-gah?*
Fever?	Fiebre?	*Fee-eh-breh?*
Insomnia?	Insomnia?	*Een-some-ne-ah?*
Skin:		
Rashes?	Sarpullido? or Erupción de la piel?	*Sahr-poo-yee-doh?* or *Ehh-roop-cion deh lah peeh-ehl?*
Skin disease?	Enfermedad de la piel?	*Ehn-fehr-meh-dad deh lah pee-ehl?*
Bumps?	Chichón/chichote?	*Chee-chohn/chee-choh-teh?*
Lesions?	Lesiones?	*Leh-see-oh-nehs?*
Itching?	Comezón?	*Koh-meh-sohn?*
Dryness?	Sequedad de su piel?	*Seh-keh-dad deh soo pee-ehl?*
Color change?	Manchas anormales en la piel?	*Mahn-chahs ah-nohr-mah-lehs ehn lah pee-ehl?*
Hair loss?	Ha perdido algo de su pelo?	*Ah pehr-dee-doh ahl-goh deh soo pah-loh?*
Head:		
Headaches?	Dolores de cabeza?	*Doh-loh-rehs deh kah-beh-sah?*
Head injury?	Un daño en la cabeza?	*Oon dah-nyoh ehn lah kah-beh-sah?*
Eyes:		
Blurred vision?	Su vista nublada?	*Soo vees-tah noo-blah-dah?*
Glasses or contact lenses?	Lentes o lentes de contacto?	*Lehn-tes o lehn-tes deh con-tac-tohs?*
Eye pain?	Dolor en los ojos?	*Doh-lohr ehn lohs oh-hoh?*
Redness in eye?	El ojo rojo?	*Ehl oh-hoh roh-hoh?*
Glaucoma?	Glaucoma?	*Glah-oo-koh-mah?*
Cataracts?	Cataratas?	*Kah-tah-rah-tahs?*
Nose and sinuses:		
Frequent colds?	La da resfriados con frecuencia?	*Leh dah rehs-free-ah-dohs kohn freh-kwen-see-ah?*
Nose bleeds easily?	Le sangra su nariz con facilidad?	*Leh sahn-grah soo nah-reehs kohn fah-see-lee-dad?*

English	Spanish	Phonetic Spanish

Throat and mouth:

Frequent sore throats?	La da con frequencia dolor de garganta?	*Leh dah kohn freh-kwen-see-ah doh-lohr deh gahr-gahn-tah?*
Hoarseness?	Ronquera?	*Rohn-keh-rah?*

Neck:

Enlarged glands?	Teine ahora glándulas agrandadas?	*Tee-eh-neh ah-oh-rah glahn-doo-lahs ah-grahn-dah-dahs?*
Stiffness?	Rígidez?	*Ree-hee-dehs?*
Have you felt any lumps in your neck?	Ha sentido alguna masa en su cuello?	*Ah sehn-tee-doh ahl-goo-nah mah-sah ehn soo kweh-yoh?*

Breasts:

Have you felt any lumps in your breasts?	Ha sentido alguna masa en su senos?	*Ah sehn-tee-doh ahl-goo-nah mah-sah ehn soo seh-nohs?*
Are your breasts or nipples painful?	Están sus senos o pezones adoloridos?	*Ehs-than soos she-nohs oh peh-soh-nehs ah-doh-loh-ree-dohs?*
Discharging?	Supurando?	*Soo-poo-rahn-doh?*

Respiratory:

Shortness of breath?	Tiene falta de aliento o aire?	*Tee-eh-neh fahl-tah deh ah-lee-ehn-toh oh ah-ee-reh?*
Cough?	Tiene tos?	*Tee-eh-neh tohs?*
Sputum?	Tiene flema en la garganta?	*Tee-eh-neh fleh-mah ehn lah gahr-gahn-tah?*
Is the color . . .	Es la flema . . .	*Ehs lah fleh-mah . . .*
Clear?	Clara?	*Klah-rah?*
Yellow?	Amarilla?	*Ah-mah-ree-yah?*
White?	Blanca?	*Blahn-kah?*
Green?	Verde?	*Vehr-deh?*
Coughed up blood?	Ha tocído sangre?	*Ah toh-see-doh sahn-greh?*
Wheezing?	Silbido de asma?	*Seel-bee-doh deh ahs-mah?*
Asthma?	Asma?	*Ahs-mah?*
Bronchitis?	Bronquitis?	*Brohn-kee-tees?*
Emphysema?	Enfisema?	*Ehn-fee-seh-mah?*
Pneumonia?	Neumonia?	*Neh-oo-moh-nee-ah?*
Tuberculosis?	Tuberculosis?	*Too-behr-koo-loh-sees?*

Cardiac:

Chest pain?	Tiene dolor en el pecho?	*Tee-eh-neh doh-lohr ehn ehl peh-choh?*
Hypertension?	Presión alta?	*Preh-see-ohn ahl-tah?*
Rheumatic fever?	Fiebre reumatica?	*Fee-eh-breh reh-oo-mah-tee-kah?*
Heart murmurs?	Murmullos del corazón?	*Moor-moo-yohs dehl koh-rah-sohn?*
Palpitations?	Tiene palpitaciones?	*Tee-eh-neh pahl-pee-tah-see-oh-nehs?*
Swollen ankles?	Tiene tobillos hinchados?	*Toh-bee-yohs een-chah-dohs?*

Gastrointestinal:

Trouble swallowing?	Tiene dificultad al tragar?	*Tee-eh-neh dee-fee-kool-tad ahl trah-gahr?*
Appetite changed?	Le ha cambiado su apetito?	*Leh ah kahm-bee-ah-doh soo ah-peh-tee-toh?*

English	Spanish	Phonetic Spanish
Nausea?	Nausea?	*Nah-oo-seh-ah?*
Vomiting?	Vomitos?	*Voh-mee-tohs?*
Vomiting blood?	Vómitos de sangre?	*Voh-mee-tohs deh sahn-greh?*
Indigestion?	Indigestión?	*Een-dee-hehs-tee-ohn?*
Abdominal pain? Where?	Le dan dolores en el abdómen? Dónde?	*Leh dahn doh-loh-rehs ehn ehl ab-doh-mehn? Dohn-deh?*
Liver problem?	Problema de higado?	*Proh-bleh-mah deh ee-gah-doh?*

Bowel movements:

Change in color and size of stools?	Cambio de color y forma del excremento?	*Kahn-bee-oh deh koh-lohr ee fohr-mah ehl egs-kreh-mehn-toh?*
Change in bowel habits?	Cambio en su defecación habitual?	*Kahm-bee-oh ehn soo deh-feh-keh-see-ohn ah-bee-too-ahl?*
Bloody stools?	Excrementos sanguíneos?	*Egs-kreh-mehn-tohs sahn-gee-neh-ohs?*
Black tarry stools?	Excremento color alquitrán Negro?	*Egs-kreh-mehn-toh koh-lohr-ahl-kee-trahn neh-groh?*
Hemorrhoids?	Hemorroides?	*Eh-moh-roy-dehs?*
Constipation?	Estreñimiento?	*Ehs-trh-nyee-mee-ehn-toh?*
Diarrhea?	Diarrea?	*Dee-ah-rheh-ah?*

Urinary:

Do you urinate often?	Orina con frequencia?	*Oh-ree-nah kohn freh-kwehn-see-ah?*
Do you have pain or burning with urination?	Tiene usted dolor o ardor cuándo orina?	*Tee-eh-neh oos-twhd doh-lohr oh ahr-dohr kwahn-doh oh-ree-nah?*
Do you get up at night to urinate?	Se levanta en la noche a orinar?	*Seh leh-vahn-tah ehn lah noh-cheh ah oh-ree-nahr?*
Do you have blood in your urine?	Tiene sangre en su orina?	*Tee-eh-neh sahn-greh ehn soo oh-ree-nah?*
Have you had a bladder infection?	Ha tenido alguna vez una infección en la vejiga?	*Ah the-nee-doh ahl-goo-nah vehs oo-nah een-feg-see-ohn ehn lah veh-hee-gah?*
Kidney infection?	Infección de los riñones?	*Een-feg-see-ohn deh lohs ree-nyoh-nehs?*
Prostatitis?	Inflamación del próstata?	*Een-flah-mah-see-ohn dehl prohs-tah-tah?*

Genital, male:

Have you had . . .	Alguna vez ha tenido . . .	*Ahl-goo-nah vehs ah the-nee-doh . . .*
Gonorrhea?	Gonorrhoea?	*Go-noh-rheh-ah?*
Herpes?	Herpes?	*Hehr-pehs?*
Syphilis?	Sifilis?	*See-fee-lees?*
Do you have pain in your testicles?	Tiene dolor en los testículos?	*Tee-eh-neh doh-lohr ehn ohs tehs-tee-koo-lohs?*
Do you have discharge from your penis?	Tiene supuración del pene?	*Tee-eh-neh soo-poo-rah-see-ohn dehl peh-neh?*

Genital, female:

Have you had . . .	Alguna vez ha tenido . . .	*Ahl-goo-nah vehs ah the-nee-doh . . .*
Gonorrhea?	Gonorrhea?	*Go-noh-rheh-ah?*
Herpes?	Herpes?	*Hehr-pehs?*
Syphilis?	Sifilis?	*See-fee-lees?*
How old were you when you started your period?	Que edad tenía cuándo empezó la regla?	*Keh eh-dad the-nee-ah kwahn-doh ehm-peh-soh lah reh-gla?*
Are your periods regular?	Son sus reglas regulares?	*Sohn soos reh-glahs reh-goo-lah-rehs?*
When was your last period?	Cuándo fue su última regla?	*Kwahn-doh fweh soo ool-tee-mah reh-glah?*

English	Spanish	Phonetic Spanish
How many times have you been pregnant?	Cuántas veces ha estado embarazada?	*Kwahn-tahs veh-sehs ah ehs-tah-doh ehm-bah-rah-sah-dah?*
Miscarriage?	Malparto?	*Mahl-pahr-toh?*
Abortion?	Aborto voluntario?	*Ah-bohr-toh voh-loon-tah-ree-oh?*
How many children do you have?	Cuántos niños tiene?	*Kwahn-tohs nee-nyohs tee-eh-neh?*

Peripheral vascular:

Leg cramps?	Calambres en la pierna?	*Kah-lahm-brehs ehn lah pee-ehr-nahs?*

Musculoskeletal:

Do you have muscle or joint pains?	Tiene dolor múscular o en coyunturas?	*Tee-eh-neh doh-lohr moos-koo-lahr oh ehn koh-yoon-too-rahs?*

Neurologic:

Fainting?	Desmayos?	*Dehs-mah-yhohs?*
Seizures?	Ataques epilépticos?	*Ah-tah-kehs eh-pee-lep-tee-kohs?*
Weakness?	Debilidad?	*Deh-bee-lee-dad?*
Paralysis?	Parálisis?	*Pah-rah-lee-sees?*
Tremors?	Temblores?	*Tehm-bloh-rehs?*

Hematologic:

Do you have anemia?	Tiene anemia?	*Tee-eh-neh ah-neh-mee-ah?*
Easy bruising or bleeding?	Usted magúlla o sangra con facilidad?	*Oos-ted mah-goo-yah oh sanh-grah kohn fah-see-lee-dad?*

Endocrine:

Thyroid problem?	Problema de tiroide?	*Proh-bleh-mah deh tee-roy-deh?*
Heat or cold intolerance?	Tiene intolerancia al calor o frio?	*Tee-eh-neh een-toh-leh-rahn-see-ah ahl kah-lohr oh free-oh?*
Diabetes?	Diabetes?	*Dee-ah-beh-tehs?*

Psychiatric:

Do you have depression?	Tiene depresión?	*Tee-eh-neh deh-preh-see-ohn?*
Any suicidal ideation?	Tiene pensamientos de suicidio?	*Tee-eh-neh pehn-sah-mee-ehn-tohs deh swee-see-dee-oh?*
Memory loss?	Tiene pérdida de memoria?	*Tee-eh-neh pehr-dee-dah deh meh-moh-ree-ah?*

PHYSICAL EXAMINATION COMMANDS

English	Spanish	Phonetic Spanish
I am going to examine you.	Voy a examinarte.	*Voy ah ehx-ah-mee-nahr-teh.*
Open your mouth.	Abre la boca.	*Ah-breh lah boh-kah.*
Say, "ahh."	Di "aaa."	*Dee ah-ah-ah.*
I am going to listen to your heart.	Voy a escuchar el corazón.	*Voy ah ehs-koo-chahr ehl koh-rah-sohn.*
Don't talk.	No hable.	*Noh ah-bleh.*
Breathe.	Respire.	*Rehs-pee-reh.*
Take a deep breath.	Respira hondo.	*Rehs-pee-rah ohn-doh.*

English	Spanish	Phonetic Spanish
Again.	Otra vez.	*Oh-trah behs.*
Please lie down here.	Por favor acuéstese aquí.	*Pohr fah-vohr ah-kwehs-teh-seh ah-kee.*
Tell me if you feel any pain when I press.	Dígame sí siente algún dolor cuándo empujo.	*Dee-gah-meh see see-ehn-teh ahl-goon doh-lohr kwahn-doh ehm-poo-hoh.*
Does it hurt here?	Le duele aquí?	*Leh dweh-leh ah-kee?*
Does it hurt when I let go?	Le duele cuándo le suelto?	*Leh dweh-leh kwahn-doh leh swehl-toh?*

Index

Note: Page numbers with an *f* indicate figures; those with a *t* indicate tables.